Motor Control

Motor Control

Edited by

Alexander A. Gydikov,
Nikolas T. Tankov,
and Dimiter S. Kosarov

Laboratory of Motor Control
Institute of Physiology
Bulgarian Academy of Sciences
Sofia, Bulgaria

SPRINGER SCIENCE+BUSINESS MEDIA, LLC

Library of Congress Cataloging in Publication Data

International Symposium on Motor Control, 2d, Zlatni Pȳasŭtsi, Bulgaria, 1973.
   Motor control.

   Selected papers from the International Union of Physiological Sciences symposium.
   Includes bibliographies.
   1. Neuromuscular transmission—Congresses. 2. Muscular sense—Congresses.
3. Motor ability—Congresses. I. Gidikov, Aleksandŭr A., ed. II. Tankov, Nikolas T.,
ed. III. Kosarov, Dimiter S., ed. IV. International Union of Physiological Sciences.
V. Title. [DNLM: 1. Motor activity—Congresses. W3 IN91985 1973m / WE103
1601 1973m]
QP369.I57   1973   599'.01'852   73-19722

ISBN 978-1-4613-4504-6   ISBN 978-1-4613-4502-2 (eBook)
DOI 10.1007/978-1-4613-4502-2

*Selected papers from the Second International Symposium on
Motor Control held at "Zlatni Pyassatsi" near Varna, Bulgaria,
October 3-7, 1973.*

© 1973 Springer Science+Business Media New York
Originally published by Plenum Press, New York in 1973
Softcover reprint of the hardcover 1st edition 1973

A Division of Plenum Publishing Corporation
227 West 17th Street, New York, N.Y. 10011

United Kingdom edition published by Plenum Press, London
A Division of Plenum Publishing Company
Davis House (4th Floor), 8 Scrubs Lane, Harlesden, London, NW10 6SE, England

P R E F A C E

The present volume contains selected papers reported at the Second International Symposium on Motor
Control held from 3rd to 7th October in the sea resort
"Zlatni Pyassatsi" near Varna, Bulgaria. The symposium
was held as a regional meeting of IUPS (International
Union of Physiological Sciences) and was aimed at extending the relations between the physiologists working
in the field of motor control from East Europe and their
colleagues from the other parts of the world. The symposium was attended by 143 scientists from 20 countries.
101 papers were presented. To include all papers in a
volume was difficult to realize in practice and perhaps
not necessary at all. Therefore, we gladly accepted the
offer of Plenum Publishing Corporation to publish selected papers.

The scientific program of the symposium included
the following topics: Muscle as a link in the motor control system. 2. Motor units. 3. Proprioception. 4. Spinal mechanisms of motor control. 5. Supraspinal mechanisms of motor control. 6. Tremor, posture and locomotion. 7. Eye-movement control. 8. Tracking movements.

The selecting of papers to be included in the
present volume turned out to be a very hard mission.
We were happy in the first place to carry the opening
lecture of R. Granit "Muscle sensitivity and proprioception in the motor control". We wanted also to in-
corporate all the invited papers but unfortunately we
failed to do that for some of them had already been
submitted for publishing elsewhere. Some other papers
have been included instead and when selecting the latter we had in view the following principles: 1. To present an over-all portrayal of the research being done in
the laboratories from East Europe whose scientific production enjoys but slighter popularity in the West because of the language barrier. 2. To present as fully

as possible the topics of the symposium. 3. To give the volume an all round and completed appearance. I would like to emphasize here that many of the papers not included in the present volume were very interesting and original, which we should have gladly incorporated had an opportunity been afforded.

The extreme complexity and perfection of the motor control system, particularly in the mammalians and man, is beyond doubt. Despite the achievements in the physiology of movements since the time of Leonardo da Vinci till our days and especially in recent decades, we are far from the full understanding of the mechanisms through which the complex algorithm of control in the motor system is effectuated. Physiology is still remaining in the stage of studying mainly the neurophysiological basis of motor control. But in the conventional neurophysiological studies one becomes ever more faced with the urgent need of understanding how in fact the subsystems in the complex hierarchical structure ensuring the motor control and the system as a whole are operating, which of the features investigated of the different elements and relationships are significant since they are manifested in the working range under normal physiological conditions, and which of them are not significant because they are not manifested in this range. In other words, study of the motor control system as a whole under normal conditions is now on the agenda. However, it is really a mistake to oppose this systematic approach to the conventional neurophysiological investigations. Study of the system without an entire knowledge of its elements and relationships is impossible. On the other hand, the conventional methods, subjects and approaches have to be perfected and must organically include the systematic approach.

All these concepts were considered when making the scientific program of the Second International Symposium on Motor Control and the selected papers reflect to some extent the program.

I wish to express my thanks to the Council of IUPS for the financial support and encouragement in the planning and execution of the symposium. I am grateful to Dr. I. Mezan for his editorial assistance with the language. I am particularly indebted also to Plenum Publishing Corporation for the publishing of this volume.

Prof. A.A. Gydikov, M.D.

CONTENTS

CONTRIBUTORS

Radmila Anastasijević, C.Sc.
    Institute for Medical Research, Belgrade, Yugoslavia
Lajos Ángyán
    Institute of Physiology, University Medical School
    of Pecs, Pecs, Hungary
J. Czarkowska
    Department of Neurophysiology, Nencki Institute of
    Experimental Biology, Polish Academy of Sciences,
    Warsaw, Poland
Nadezhda I. Draganova
    Laboratory of Applied Neurophysiology and Psycho-
    physiology, Research Institute for Work Hygiene
    and Labor Protection, Sofia, Bulgaria
Stefan S. Dunev
    Laboratory of Applied Neurophysiology and Psycho-
    physiology, Research Institute for Work Hygiene
    and Labor Protection, Sofia, Bulgaria
Sergey V. Fomin, D.Sc.
    Professor, Faculty of Mechanics and Mathematics,
    State University of Moscow, Moscow, USSR
G. Gantchev
    Laboratory of Applied Neurophysiology and Psycho-
    physiology, Research Institute for Work Hygiene
    and Labor Protection, Sofia, Bulgaria
Velitchko A. Gatev, M.D.
    Senior Research Associate, Department of Develop-
    mental Physiology, Research Institute of Pediatrics,
    Sofia, Bulgaria
Teresa Gòrska
    Adiunkt, Department of Neurophysiology, Nencki In-
    stitute of Experimental Biology, Polish Academy of
    Sciences, Warsaw, Poland
Ragnar Granit
    Professor, The Nobel Institute for Neurophysiology,
    Karolinska Institutet, Stockholm, Sweden

Sten Grillner
        Associate Professor, Department of Physiology,
        University of Göteborg, Göteborg, Sweden
Otto-Joachim Grüsser, M.D.
        Professor, Neurophysiology Section, Institute of
        Physiology, Freie Universität Berlin, West Berlin
Victor S. Gurfinkel, M.D.
        Professor, Laboratory of Motor Control, Institute
        of the Problems of Information Transmission, Acade-
        my of Sciences USSR, Moscow, USSR
Alexander A. Gydikov, M.D.
        Professor, Laboratory of Motor Control, Institute
        of Physiology, Bulgarian Academy of Sciences, So-
        fia, Bulgaria
Heidemarie Hohne-Zahn
        Neurophysiology Section, Institute of Physiology,
        Freie Universität Berlin, West Berlin
Saburo Homma
        Professor, Department of Physiology, School of
        Medicine, Chiba University, Chiba, Japan
Ivan A. Ivanov
        Department of Development Physiology, Research
        Institute of Pediatrics, Sofia, Bulgaria
Samia A.Jahn
        Department of Physiology, University of Khartoum,
        Sudan
K. Kanda
        Department of Physiology, School of Medicine, Chiba
        University, Chiba, Japan
Dimiter Kosarov
        Institute of Physiology, Bulgarian Academy of
        Sciences, Sofia, Bulgaria
Platon G. Kostyuk, D.Sc.
        Corresponding Member of the Acad.Sc.,Professor and
        Director, S.S. Bogomoletz Institute of Physiology,
        Academy of Sciences of Ukr.SSR, Kiev, USSR
L.Lénárd
        Institute of Physiology, University Medical School
        of Pecs, Pecs, Hungary
Kalman Lissák, Academician
        Professor and Director, Institute of Physiology,
        University Medical School of Pecs, Pecs, Hungary
K. Pellnitz
        Neurophysiology Section, Institute of Physiology,
        Freie Universität Berlin, West Berlin
Alexander I. Shapovalov, M.D.
        Professor, Laboratory of Physiology of the Nerve
        Cell, Sechenov Institute of Evolutive Physiology
        and Biochemistry, Academy of Sciences USSR, Lenin-
        grad, USSR

Mark L. Shik, D.Sc.
        Senior Research Associate, Laboratory of Motor
        Control, Institute of the Problems of Information,
        Academy of Sciences USSR, Moscow, USSR
T. I. Stillkind
        Institute of the Problems of Information Transmis-
        sion, Academy of Sciences USSR, Moscow, USSR
Åke B. Vallbo
        Associate Professor, Department of Physiology,
        University of Umeå, Umeå, Sweden
Jovan Vučo
        Senior Research Associate, Associate Professor of
        Research, Institute for Medical Research, Belgrade,
        Yugoslavia

OPENING LECTURE

MUSCLE SENSE, PROPRIOCEPTION AND THE CONTROL OF MOVEMENT

R.GRANIT[x]

From the Nobel Institute for Neurophysiology
Karolinska Institutet

Stockholm, Sweden

INTRODUCTION

The term 'kinaesthetic sense' was introduced by
Bastian (1887) who had been asked by the Council of the
Neurological Society in London to open a discussion on
the 'muscular sense', its nature and cortical localiza-
tion. His report was published in 'Brain' together with
brief contributions from leading neurologists of the day.
He defined the new term as 'sense of movement' while
Bell (1826, 1833), choosing to emphasize another aspect
of his 'muscular sense', had described it as a sense of
exertion. Later it has been variously termed sense of
force or sense of resistance.

At the time of the discussion in London it was
generally realized that a muscular sensation depended on
several types of peripheral afferents and thus was a
complex percept. It was also understood that — in Bastian's words — "the full blaze of consciousness" only
became involved in "new or unfamiliar voluntary action".
In agreement with what we believe today, Bastian also
thought that the information from the proprioceptive
organs normally is incorporated in the fabric of automatic movement as 'guides only'. The term proprioception was later coined by Sherrington reviewing this
field in Schäfer's Textbook (1900). It is less specific

[x]This study was conducted while a Fogarty Scholar-in-
Residence; Fogarty international Center, National Insti-
tutes of Health, Bethesda, Maryland 200 14, U.S.A.

than the other two, lumping together as it does the messages concerned with position, force and movement of the
limbs and separating them from the exteroceptive and in-
teroceptive senses. The early literature on the 'muscular sense' will be found reviewed in Bastian's papers
(1869, 1887).

My reason for returning to these problems - after
a perusal of old and new contributions to this field -
is that a reassessment of it is of interest, partly because some relatively unknown old observations need be
rescued from oblivion, partly because of recent important
advances in our understanding of motor control. Thus,
for instance, the gamma loop can hardly be neglected in
discussing such problems. However, in the first section
I propose to show that Bastian's choice of 'movement'
and Bell's of 'exertion' for defining muscular sensations can be well defended. They are both likely to be
referable to definite sensory endings.

THE PSYCHOPHYSICAL APPROACH

Absolute and difference thresholds rose to the front
line of interest at the time of Weber (1834, 1846) whose
rule originally was based on experiments on weight-lift-
ing. Although never ousted from the repertoire of approaches, threshold measurements nevertheless are stereo-
typed in design compared with the acts involved in movements and posture which are executed against changing
forces of loading and length variations of muscles.These
forces continuously modify the excitability of the motoneurons of the acting muscles by producing reflex responses to tension and extension. These reflexes are reasonably well known today. They may produce constant errors of execution and judgement, as pointed out by the
author (Granit, 1972) in a re-interpretation of a number
of old papers.

Psychophysics deals with sensations and aims at de-
scribing them in c.g.s. units. In this particular regard
it faces two major difficulties: (I) the fact that our
movements are based on automatic patterns layed down in
our experience, as moulded by demand and ckecked by accomplishment; this has made us thoroughly familiar with
movements within our own 'body space'; (II) that there
is redundancy of information in the messages from joints,
tendon organs, muscle spindles and skin receptors so
that removal or loss of one type of afferent input quickly is compensated. Accordingly, if a measured perceptual

response is uninfluenced by the loss of one source of
information, it is hardly possible to conclude that this
particular source under no circumstances could have contributed to it. Remaining pathways to the central inter-
preter suffice to throw sentient circuits into action.

However, the absolute threshold does indicate which
kind of end organ is likely to be the most adequate one
for a given type of stimulus. Thus the absolute threshold for movement was ascribed by Goldscheider (1898)to
the endings in the joints. His experiments were extensive
and well controlled; they have often been reviewed and
many times repeated (e.g. Laidlow and Hamilton,1937;Cleg-
horn and Darcus, 1952; Browne, Lee and Ring, 1954; Provins, 1958; and reviews by Gardner, 1950 and Howard and
Templeton, 1966). The electrophysiological studies of
impulses from endings in the joints and their central
projections (e.g. Boyd and Roberts, 1953; S.Skoglund,
1956; Mountcastle and Powell, 1959; Burgess and Clark,
1969) provide a satisfactory explanation of the threshold for movement, partly also of its dependence upon the
velocity of movement. If the criterion of measurement be
widened to include direction of movement, many other cues
are likely to contribute to this percept.

Von Frey who - wrongly, as we know today - refused
to believe in the existence of joint nerves pursued this
question of sense of direction in several papers (1917/18,
1918/19; v.Frey and Meyer, 1917/18). He found - as had
Goldscheider - the threshold increased but also more
precise when his subjects were requested to respond also
to the direction of movement. This result has been confirmed. Thus, to give an example, Cleghorn and Darcus
(1952) recorded a just perceptible movement at the elbow
joint for a displacement of 0.8^{O} while detection of its
direction required 1.8^{O} (criterion 80% correct answers).
V.Frey's arguments against joint receptors have not
stood the test of time.

The most important contribution of v.Frey dealt
with the sense of force ('Kraftsinn'), as it established
that one can judge accurately about the equality of
forces when weights are placed at different distances
from the elbow joint upon an arm encased in plaster of
Paris (v.Frey, 1913, 1914). These were the first well-
controlled attempts to measure force accurately. He also
determined weight differences by a technique of 'Schleuderung' implying that two slightly different apple-sized
weights were tossed up rhythmically some six to eight
times. Their basic weight was 800 g but they contained
a locked receptacle hiding interchangeable small weights.

Perceived differences of weight were of the order 0.5
per cent. In terms of equivalent muscle tension this was
calculated to correspond to a sensitivity of 0.25 per
cent. Such extreme accuracy presupposes at least one highly sensitive ending.

Today we know that muscle spindles are incredibly
sensitive to changes of length (Lundberg and Winsbury,
1960). The thresholds of primary spindle endings are of
the order of 4-5μ(Brown, Engberg and Matthews, 1967;
Stuart, Mosher, Gerlach and Reinking, 1970). Tamaki(1967)
studied the absolute thresholds for minimal velocities
of stretching in the triceps surae of the cat and found
spindle primaries to require 3 mm/sec while the tendon
organs needed 10 mm/sec. Both organs are stretch receptors
and so would have been slightly stretched by the falling
weight in v.Frey's experiments (small falling weight).

Renqvist (1926 a) measured the absolute threshold of
force (resistance) in the finger of three subjects after
it had been anaesthetized with an injection of 5 ml novo-
caine (with suprarenin). The finger did not feel a weight
of 20-25 g on the skin and was insensitive to small slow
movements without this load. Force or resistance was felt
with active movements for a load of about 10 g on the
finger. This was calculated to correspond to 0.5 per cent
of the maximum force per sq. cm cross section of muscle.
The need for active movements suggests spindle activation.

V.Frey's technique of 'Schleuderung' indicates that
the movement itself was ballistic, that is, a brief
twitch transferring its energy into the momentum of the
moving hand. By contrast a subsequent development of Renqvist's (1926 b) was based on the inertia ergometer of
Hill (1922) and this instrument makes use of a load that
opposes the muscle to the inertia of a mass whose reaction (in the Newtonian sense) always is equal to the
force applied to it by the muscle (Hill). This apparatus
consists of a rotating shaft loaded with concentric
weights and, in Renqvist's experiments, it was turned by
a lever in an extension-flexion movement of the arm. An
example: when the load was 9.59 kg, the forearm was made
to swing the lever at two amplitudes related as 4:2. At
the smaller amplitude the arm had to be accelerated in
order for the weight to be felt equally heavy as at the
larger amplitude. The acceleration that was required for
the percept of equality of force (resistance) proved to
be the very amount that satisfied the equation by which
force is defined as the product of mass times acceleration.

Evidently some end organ must be responsible for the preception of resistance or force which implies that Bell's sense of exertion really exists as a muscular sensation. The candidates are muscle spindles or tendon organs or both conjointly. Since muscle spindles are activated across the gamma loop by volitional impulses (see below, 'ALPHA-GAMMA LINKAGE'), these are the most likely force receptors, at least for operations requiring high sensitivity. Our perceptions then demand full attention directed to the task at hand. Even so, in spite of its astonishing accuracy, the awareness of force cannot be compared in vividness and detailed specification with impressions from major exteroceptors such as the eye and the ear. Probably sense of resistance describes it most adequately.

The two percepts of movement and of force are the only ones for which the evidence available suggests specific end organs. Other attributes of movement can be measured quite accurately but are nevertheless likely to be based on composite information. Fullerton and Cattell (1892) studied force, extent and time of movement and concluded that "extent of movements can be judged better than force, and the force better than the time" (p.158). This statement was based on extensive experimentation. However, force was not physically as accurately checked as in the experiments of v.Frey and Renqvist. Velocity of movement is a very direct impression but since most sensory endings in joints, muscle and skin are rate-sensitive, all of them are likely to contribute to this percept. If extent (displacement) were represented by one sense organ only, it would not be intermingled with duration and velocity in such a manner as virtually to disappear for maintained positions (Bloch, 1896; Paillard and Brouchon, 1968), nor would it be dependent on muscle extension in the particular way it is found to be in Loeb's illusion (Loeb, 1890). After innumerable experiences from childhood onwards displacements within the body space must be represented by well-ingrained memories producing wholly automatized acts. Woodworth (1901) analyzed 125,000 movements from the point of view of accuracy and succinctly summarized his results in the statement: "by association, the control of movement may come to depend on sensations of any sort" (p.75). There is a recent confirmation of this generalization in the findings of Marsden, Merton and Morton (1972) that anaesthesia of the skin on the thumb removes an automatic load-compensating response of flexion at the top joint.

ALPHA-GAMMA LINKAGE

It was mentioned above that the muscle spindles
have been shown to be co-activated with their muscles
also in volitional acts (Hagbarth and Vallbo, 1968, 1969;
Vallbo, 1970, 1971). The evidence is based on direct recording of spindle impulses from the nerves of human
subjects. So far it chiefly refers to the afferents of
spindle primary endings but, since these were found to
discharge during maintained contractions, it is permis-
sible to conclude that the secondary endings must also
have been activated (as to why, see Granit, 1970, Ch.IV).
Much recent experimental work goes to show that the
spindle endings project to the cerebrum and the cerebellum (see e.g. in cats, Oscarsson and Rosén, 1963;
Oscarsson, 1966; Landgren and Silfvenius, 1969; in ba-
boons, Phillips, Powell and Wiesendanger, 1971). It has
been known since 1952 (Granit and Kaada, 1952) that a
considerable number of central stations display linked
alpha-gamma output. Several long loops may exist by
which these outputs to the spindles are fed back to the
central stations.Experiments on volitional acts are of
particular interest because they serve to actualize a
physiological approach to the understanding of events
characterized by psychological terms such as 'demand'
and 'accomplishment' (Granit, 1972). Inasmuch as movements are based on central programs it is no more a question of whether or not kinaesthetic information is fed
back. Alpha-gamma linkage ensures that it always is present. Unless actively inhibited, it is bound to produce
an effect.

DEMAND AND ACCOMPLISHMENT

A volitional alpha-gamma output inevitably represents a 'demand' but the reversed statement would not hold
good; demands can be executed without evoking any volitional effort whatsoever. Thus, for instance, the respiratory centres demand that a certain volume of air be in-
haled and do so by wholly automatic alpha-gamma linkage
supported by vagal and diaphragmatic reflexes, as eluci-
dated in the cat by direct recording (Corda, Eklund and
Euler, 1965). The term 'volitional' implies an involve-
ment of consciousness, often merely as a trigger for
virtually automatic acts. The boundaries between conscious and automatic goal-directed motor acts are
fleeting. For most purposes only an operational definition of 'consciousness' is required: it is a mechanism
for selecting the wanted alpha-gamma combination from a

repertoire of familiar components. By setting up demands
the experimenter avails himself of it.

Demanded motor acts have long been studied, in particular from psychotechnical aspects as part of man-ma-
chine engineering problems. The point raised here is
that, with a circuit available which is known to be capable of expressing demand as well as of feeding information on its accomplishment back to the higher centres,
this is the one that in the first instance need be studied because it provides the physiologist with a unique
opportunity of closing the gap between his concepts and
those of psychology such as 'will', 'demand', 'expecta-
tion', 'set', 'accomplishment' in so far as such concepts
are used in the description of motor acts. In man there
is no other case available in which a feedback response
is obtained in terms of nerve impulses. The volitional
component can now be analyzed in experiments on man in
the manner of Hagbarth and Vallbo.

'Demand' as an experimental proposition is many-
facetted. One can ask for a certain amount of force, of
displacement, of velocity or acceleration in execution,
for any combination of these factors as well as for the
use of specific muscles or even motor units. 'Accomplishment' is ultimately determined by evaluation of errors
of performance. When such errors exceed a certain mag-
nitude the subject consciously registers a 'mismatch'
between his intentions and their execution. There are
also constant errors or illusions which the subject is
unaware of. I have discussed them elsewhere (Granit,
1972) inasmuch as they are likely to be caused by errors
of feedback in the shape of spindle reflexes. Considerable interest now attaches to experiments planned to
elucidate — by direct recording   the role of feedback
in determining errors of performance.

OPENING THE 'BLACK BOX' OF PROPRIOCEPTIVE CONTROL

The psychologist in his stimulus-response studies
and the psychotechnically interested engineer share a
common interest in the variance encountered in different
arrangements of an experiment. They are alike also in
being satisfied by attributing the actual processes involved to a 'black box' whose inside is and always will
remain closed. However, the psychologist must be credit-
ed with less willingness than the engineer to discuss
tracking experiments solely as simple servo-systems
across an error-actuated human operator (Adams, 1961).

He is aware of complications such as motivation, expecta-
tion and anticipation (e.g.Gibbs, 1954; Adams and Creamer, 1962).

The task of the physiologist is to remove the lid
of the 'black box' and take a peep at the inside. He does
this by intercepting in- and outgoing messages at many
different sites in the nervous system, timing them accurately at those sites and measuring them quantitatively.
By such procedures he should in the end be able to delineate the features of the organization responsible for
movement.

Some examples of recent experiments will serve to
illustrate means of opening the black box from the physiological end. The direct-recording technique of Evarts
(1966, 1967) in which a monkey is trained to execute an
extension-flexion movement at the wrist and is rewarded
for specific demands (speed, resistance, displacement
etc.) has shown that several central sites act to anti-
cipate such movements or are concomitantly active. His
work and that of Humphrey, Schmidt and Thompson (1970)
deals with cortical neurons sending their messages along
the pyramidal tract. By this technique Thach (1970) has
found cerebellar neurons and DeLong (1971) pallidal neurons participating in such motor acts. For these simple
movements the reverberation of the commands within the
central nervous system may seem greater than might have
been expected, even when considering that some of the
messages could refer to postural adjustments accompanying movement.

The movement studied by the technique of Evarts is
a volitional act for which the monkey has been trained.
From the work of Phillips (1969) much is known about
cortical stimulation and its effect upon motoneurons belonging to the hand of the baboon. Supplementary evidence
could be obtained by his technique, extended to testing
other sites in the brain, to elucidate how, or if at all,
movements elicited from the motor cortex by electrical
stimulation differ in their central distribution from
their volitional counterparts. It seems likely that the
neuronal organization associated with a movement consists of co-operating prime movers as well as of sites
representing various controls (visual, vestibular) to
which information is dispatched because such sites are
in need of knowing that a movement is afoot. One can
easily imagine that if sensory messages suddenly begin
to pour in to them from joints, skin, tendons and muscles, the context in which this happens need be known in

order to prevent meaningless responses.

It will not always be easy to differentiate between actual prime movers (motor cortex, basal ganglia) and sites in need of information, unless it follows straight away from accurate timing of the message at these sites. The pathology of movement and the study of ablations and other selective lesions will continue to provide a lead. Destruction of prime movers, phasic or tonic, would be likely to leave permanent defects of movement or posture while compensation should be expected if centres are lost that are less directly concerned with the muscular acts.

An instructive case of a demand reflected by alpha-gamma linkage has been published by Vallbo (1971). By the direct-recording technique applied to a human subject he has shown that a greater volitional contraction pro-duces a correspondingly greater rate of spindle discharge. Limits for quantification of this experiment seem to be set by the difficulty of maintaining the tip of the record-ing electrode in position in the fibre that it has isolat-ed. However, since most movements are upheld by several muscles, sequentially in different states of activity, closeness of alpha-gamma co-activation could possibly be checked by locating spindles belonging to several par-ticipants in a motor act. To illustrate what is meant I have taken the description of the relatively simple move-ment of opening the closed fist from the classical work of Duchenne (1867, English translation 1949):

"In effect, the extensors of the fingers (the com-mon and the proprius) extend only the proximal phalanges. The interossei which extend the two terminal phalanges must contract synergistically with the preceding muscles to produce complete extension of the three phalanges. On the other hand, the interossei cannot extend the two distal phalanges without simultaneously producing flexion of the proximal phalanges. Fortunately this flexion is neutralized by a reversed action of the ex-tensors. Finally, as the extensors of the fingers pull simultaneously into extension the wrist and the phal-anges, the volar muscles enter into synergic action in direct proportion to the force of the extensors of the fingers. Then the hand can be held in extension in line with the forearm, without the participation of the pro-per extensors of the wrist (the extensor carpi radialis and the extensor carpi ulnaris" (pp. 550-551).

It is impossible in these brief comments on prospects

for work on motor control and proprioception to scan the
extensive repertoire of possible approaches to these problems. The interest has been centered on man as a subject
in psycho-physiological experiments and consequently also
on the highly corticalized monkey. When it has been pointed out that psychological concepts can be translated into
physiological experiments based on direct recording, it
is perhaps necessary to add a reservation. I have not ad-
vocated a psycho-physiology of the kind that, for instance, connects electroencephalographic observations on
'brain waves' to 'attention', 'expectancy' etc. This is
pure phenomenology that does not carry understanding much
beyond our common conviction that something happens in
the brain whenever a psychological state or concept can
be somehow defined. My intention has been to emphasize
that we now possess such means of analyzing the neural
organization of motor acts as are applicable also to
those acts that are based on instructions defined in
psychological terms.

REFERENCES

ADAMS, J.A. (1961). Human tracking behaviour. Psychol.
   Rev. 58; 55-79.
ADAMS, J.A. & CREAMER, L.R. (1962). Proprioception
   variables as determiners of anticipatory timing be-
   haviour. Human factors 4: 217-222.
BASTIAN, Ch. (1869). On the "muscular sense" and on the
   physiology of thinking. Brit.Med.J. (May issues and
   June 5th issue)
BASTIAN, Ch. (1887). The "muscular sense"; its nature
   and cortical localisation. Brain 10: 1-89.
BELL, Ch. (1826). On the nervous circle which connects
   the voluntary muscles with the brain. Phil.Trans.Roy.
   Soc., pp. 163-173.
BELL, Ch. (1833). The Hand, 5th edn. 1855. London:
   John Murray.
BLOCH, A.-M. (1896). Note apropos de la communication
   de M.Féré (Expériences relatives à la notion de posi-
   tion). C.R.Soc.Biol. 48: 81-82.
BOYD, I.A. & ROBERTS, T.D.M. (1953). Proprioceptive
   discharges from stretch-receptors in the knee-joint of
   the cat. J.Physiol.(Lond.) 122: 38-58
BROWN, M.C., ENGBERG, I. & MATTHEWS, P.B.C. (1967).
   The relative sensitivity to vibration of muscle re-
   ceptors of the cat. J.Physiol.(Lond.) 192: 773-800.
BROWNE, K., LEE, J. & RING, P.A. (1954). The sensation
   of passive movement at the metatarso-phalangeal joint
   of the great toe in man. J.Physiol.(Lond.)126:448-458.

BURGESS, P.R. & CLARK, F.J. (1969). Characteristics of
  knee joint receptors in the cat. J.Physiol.(Lond.)
  203: 317-335.
CLEGHORN, T.E. & DARCUS, H.D. (1952). The sensitivity
  to passive movement of the human elbow joint. Quart.
  J.exp.Psychol. 4: 66-77.
CORDA, M., EKLUND, G. & EULER, C.v. (1965). External
  intercostal and phrenic α motor responses to changes
  in respiratory load. Acta physiol.scand. 63: 391-400.
DeLONG, M.R. (1971). Activity of pallidal neurons during movement. J.Neurophysiol. 34: 414-427.
DUCHENNE, G.B. (1867). Physiologie des Mouvements. Paris:
  Ballière & fils. Engl.translation by E.B.Kaplan, Physiology of Motion. Philadelphia: J.B.Lippincott, 1949.
EVARTS, E.V. (1966). Pyramidal tract activity associated
  with a conditioned hand movement in the monkey. J.Neuro-
  physiol. 29: 1011-1027.
EVARTS, E.V. (1967). Representation of movements and
  muscles by pyramidal tract neurons of the precentral
  motor cortex. In Neurophysiological Basis of Normal and
  Abnormal Motor Activities, ed. M.D.YAHR & D.PURPURA,
  pp. 215-251. Hewlett: Raven Press.
FREY, M.v. (1913). Studien über den Kraftsinn. Zt.Biol.
  63: 129-154.
FREY, M.v. (1914). Die Vergleichung von Gewichten mit
  Hilfe des Kraftsins. Zt. Biol. 65: 203-224.
FREY, M.v. (1917/18). Über Bewegungswahrnemungen und Be-
  wegungen in resezierten und in anästhetischen Gelenken.
  Zt. Biol. 68: 339-350.
FREY, M.v. (1918/19). Weitere Beobachtungen über die
  Wahrnehmung von Bewegungen nach Gelenkresektion. Zt.
  Biol. 69: 322-330.
FREY, M.v. & MEYER, O.B. (1917/18). Versuche über die
  Wahrnehmung geführter Bewegungen. Zt.Biol.68: 301-338.
FULLERTON, G.S. & CATTELL, J.McK. (1892). On the Per-
  ception of Small Differences. Philadelphia: Univ.Penn-
  sylvania Press.
GARDNER, E. (1950). Physiology of movable joints. Phy-
  siol.Rev. 30: 127-176.
GIBBS, O.B. (1954). The continuous regulation of skilled
  response by kinaesthetic feed back. Brit.J.Psychol.
  45: 24-39.
GOLDSCHEIDER, A. (1898). Gesammelte Abhandlungen,II,
  Physiologie des Muskelsinnes. Leipzig: Barth.
GRANIT, R. (1970). The Basis of Motor Control. London:
  Academic Press.
GRANIT, R. (1972). Constant errors in the execution and
  appreciation of movement. Brain. In course of publica-
  tion.
GRANIT, R. & KAADA, B.R. (1952). Influence of stimula-

tion of central nervous structures on muscle spindles
in cat. Acta physiol.scand. 27: 130-160.

HAGBARTH, K.-E. & VALLBO, Å.B. (1968). Discharge characteristics of human muscular afferents during muscle
stretch and contraction. Exp.Neurol. 22: 674-694.

HAGBARTH, K.-E. & VALLBO, Å.B. (1969). Single unit recordings from muscle nerves in human subjects. Acta
physiol.scand. 76: 321-334.

HILL, A.V. (1922). The maximum work and mechanical efficiency of human muscles and their most economical
speed. J.Physiol.(Lond.) 56: 19-41.

HOWARD, I.P. & TEMPLETON, W.B. (1966). Human Spatial
Orientation. London, New York: Wiley & Sohn.

HUMPHREY, D.R., SCHMIDT, E.M. & THOMPSON, W.O. (1970).
Predicting measures of motor performance from multiple
cortical spike trains. Science. 170: 758-762.

LAIDLAW, R.W. & HAMILTON, M.A. (1937). The quantitative
measurement of apperception of passive movements.
Bull.Neurol.Inst. New York 6: 145-153.

LANDGREN, S. & SILFVENIUS, H. (1969). Projection to
cerebral cortex of Group I muscle afferents from the
cat's hindlimb. J.Physiol.(Lond.) 200: 353-372.

LOEB; J. (1890). Untersuchungen über die Orientierung
im Fühlraum der Hand und im Blickraum. Pflügers Arch.
46: 1-45.

LUNDBERG, A. & WINSBURY, G. (1960). Selective adequate
activation of large afferents from muscle spindles
and Golgi tendon organs. Acta physiol.scand. 49: 155-
164.

MARSDEN, C.D., MERTON, P.A. & MORTON, H.B. (1972).
Changes in loop gain with force in the human muscle
servo. J.Physiol.(Lond.) 222: 32-34P.

MOUNTCASTLE, V.B. & POWELL, T.P.S. (1959). Central
nervous mechanisms subserving position sense and kine-
sthesis. Bull.Johns Hopk. Hosp. 105: 173-200.

OSCARSSON, O. (1966). The projection of Group I muscle
afferents to the cat cerebral cortex. In Muscular
Afferents and Motor Control. Nobel Symp. I., ed. R.
GRANIT, pp. 307-316. Stockholm: Almqvist & Wiksell.

OSCARSSON, O. & ROSEN, I. (1963). Projection to cerebral
cortex of large muscle spindle afferents in forelimb
nerves of the cat. J.Physiol.(Lond.) 169: 924-945.

PAILLARD, J. & BROUCHON, M. (1968). Active and passive
movement in the calibration of position sense. In
The Neurophysiology of Spatially Oriented Behaviour,
ed. S.J. FREEDMAN, pp. 37-55. Homewood, Ill.: Dorsey
Press.

PHILLIPS, C.G. (1969). Motor apparatus of the baboon's
hand. The Ferrier Lecture. Proc.Roy.Soc.,B. 173:
141-174.

PHILLIPS, C.G., POWELL, T.P.S. & WIESENDANGER, M. (1971).
  Projection from low-threshold muscle afferents of hand
  and forearm to area 3a of baboon's cortex. J.Physiol.
  (Lond.) 217: 419-446.
PROVINS, K.A. (1958). The effect of peripheral nerve
  block on the appreciation and execution of finger movements. J.Physiol.(Lond.) 143: 55-67.
RENQVIST, Y. (1926a). Ueber die Reizschwelle der Kraft-
  empfindungen. Zt.Biol. 85: 391-405.
RENQVIST, Y. (1926b). Über den Bewegungswahrnehmungen
  zugrunde liegenden Reize. Skand.Arch.Physiol. 50:
  58-96.
SHERRINGTON, C.S. (1900). The muscular sense. In Schäfer's Text-book of Physiology, II, pp. 1002-1025.
  Edinburgh and London: Pentland.
SKOGLUND, S. (1956). Anatomical and physiological
  studies of knee joint innervation in the cat. Acta
  physiol.scand. 36: Suppl. 124.
STUART, G., MOSHER, C.G., GERLACH, R.L. & REINKING, R.M.
  (1970). Selective activation of Ia afferents by transient muscle stretch. Exp.Brain Res. 10: 477-487.
TAMAKI, T. (1967). Muscle spindle and tendon organ discharges during phasic muscle stretching. J.Chiba Med.
  Soc. 43: 35-36.
THACH, W.T. (1970). Discharge of cerebellar neurons related to two maintained postures and to prompt movements. I & II. J.Neurophysiol. 33: 527-547.
VALLBO, Å.B. (1970). Slowly adapting muscle receptors
  in man. Acta physiol.scand. 78: 315-333.
VALLBO, Å.B. (1971). Muscle spindle responses at the
  onset of isometric voluntary contraction in man. Time
  differences between fusimotor and skeletomotor effects.
  J.Physiol.(Lond.) 218: 405-531.
WEBER, E.H. (1834). De pulsu resorptione, auditu et
  tactu annotationes. Anat. et physiol. Leipzig pp.
  135, 137. Quoted in Weber (1846).
WEBER, E.H. (1846). Der Tastsinn und das Gemeingefühl.
  In Wagner's Handwörterbuch d.Physiologie 3: 481-588.
WOODWORTH, R.S. (1901). On the voluntary control of
  movement. Psychol.Rev. 8: 350-359.

THE ENCODING OF THE RECEPTOR POTENTIAL INTO IMPULSE

PATTERNS OF MUSCLE SPINDLE AFFERENTS OF CATS

O.-J.GRÜSSER, Heidemarie HOHNE-ZAHN, Samia A.
JAHN[x] and K.PELLNITZ

From the Neurophysiology Section, Institute of
Physiology , Freie Universität Berlin
Berlin (West)

INTRODUCTION

The muscle spindle receptors are activated if their
aequatorial region is stretched above the threshold value.
The response of the receptor potential of muscle spindle
afferents in deefferented muscles probably depends on the
muscle length according to a second order linear differential equation. The non-linear components observed in the
responses of afferent fibres (impulse patterns) might be
caused by three factors:

(1) A possible non-linear transmission along the
    chain: stimulus apparatus-extrafusal muscle -
    muscle spindle.
(2) Non-linear mechanical properties of the muscle
    spindle.
(3) Non-linear components of the encoder process,
    i.e. a non-linear transformation of the slow
    receptor potential of the receptive fiber en-
    dings into the sequence of impulses conducted
    along the axon

---

[x]University of Khartoum, Sudan, Department of
 Physiology, visiting scientist at the Institute of
 Physiology, Berlin (West), Summer 1970

The present report deals with properties of the impulse encoder. In preceding publications it was demonstrated that the non-linearity of the responses of muscle
spindle afferents observed with sinusoidal stretching of
the gastrocnemius muscles of cats might be explained
mainly by the non-linearity of the threshold mechanisms
of the encoder process (Grüsser and Thiele, 1968; Eysel
and Grüsser, 1970):

(a) The threshold Θ_t of the encoder rises after each
single impulse virtually to ∞ and is assumed to decay as
a hyperbolic function of time :

$$\Theta_t = \frac{k^*}{t} + \Theta_0 \quad [mV] \tag{1}$$

whereby $t > 0$. Whenever the receptor membrane potential
at the encoder side exceeds Θ_t , an impulse is discharged.
Θ_0 is the basic threshold level.

Eq. (1) introduces a hysteresis into the relationship between the amplitude of the receptor potential and
the impulse sequence, if the change of the amplitude of
the receptor potential is considerably fast in comparison
to the constant k^*. Eq. (1), however, predicts the ap-
proximate linear relationship between neuronal impulse
rate and muscle length found for a steady stretch. Of
course, it is difficult to conceive of a physiological
process which follows a hyperbolic function. The experimental data can also be approximated by a set of 2 or 3
exponential functions having different time constants. A
simple exponential function, however, is insufficient for
the quantitative description of the experimental data.
Therefore, we have chosen eq. (1) as one of the simplest
formal descriptions of the threshold of the encoder process Θ_t during the relative refractory period.

(b) If the receptor potential is considerably above
Θ_0 , the threshold decay after a single impulse depends
not only on eq. (1) but also on the intervals of n preceding impulses. One finds a summation of "remaining" threshold elevations, caused by the preceding impulses. Hence,
one can write instead of eq. (1):

$$\Theta_t = \sum_{j=1}^{j=n} \frac{k^*}{t-t_j} \cdot H(t-t_j) + \Theta_0 - \alpha(t) \quad [mV] \tag{2}$$

$t_j > 0$, whereby $\alpha(t)$ is a function which prevents the divergence of the sum and $H(t-t_j)$ is the unit step function:

$$H(t) = \begin{Bmatrix} 1, t > 0 \\ 0, t < 0 \end{Bmatrix}$$

With the limitation $n < 6$, the response of primary and secondary muscle spindle afferents of the cat's gastrocnemius muscle to sinusoidal stimulation could be simulated fairly well by a digital computer model of eq. (2), whereby the correcting function $\alpha(t)$ could be discarded ($\alpha(t) = 0$) (Eysel, 1971).

Eq. (2) further predicts a sequential dependence of successive impulse intervals in the response pattern of the muscle spindle afferents. Such a sequential dependence was indeed found. Significant positive or negative, serial correlation coefficients of first and higher order and a Markov-chain of first and second order were discovered for the impulse pattern of muscle spindle afferents elicited by mechanical stimuli (Eysel and Grüsser, 1970). The results of the experiments described in the present report support the postulate of the temporal summation of remaining threshold elevations. It is well-known since many years (c.f. the review by P.B.C. Matthews, 1964) that a steady-state, mechanical stimulation elicits in primary and secondary muscle spindle afferents a very regular, impulse pattern. It was predictable from eq. (2) that extra impulses, added to such a regular impulse train that is caused by a constant receptor potential, would lead to a temporal increase of the impulse intervals following the additional impulses.

These extra impulses were elicited in our experiments by antidromic electrical stimulation of the isolated afferent fiber. The stimulus was triggered by one of the "regular" action potentials, whereby the delay Δt between triggering action potentials and antidromic stimulus was changed systematically. Eq. (2) predicts that the shorter the delay Δt between the triggering action potential and the antidromic stimulus, the longer the increase of the first impulse interval I_1 after the additional antidromic impulse (fig. 2).

This method of antidromic stimulation was introduced into the muscle spindle physiology by B.H.C. Matthews (1931, 1933). He found a "reset" of the impulse train

after an antidromic impulse in frog muscle spindle afferents. In cat muscle spindle afferents, in addition to
the reset of the impulse train, the first impulse interval after the descending additional impulses was
longer, the shorter Δt. Matthews has mentioned also that
I_1 increased as the number of impulses in an antidromic
impulse train was increased. The latter observation was
further investigated by Paintal (1959a), who showed
that I_1 increases with the frequency and the duration of
the antidromic impulse train. The goal of the present
investigation was to obtain sufficient quantitative data
to test the predictions of eq. (2), i.e. to test whether the non-linear properties of the impulse encoder of
the receptor potential might be considered to be a main
source of the non-linear overall transfer property of
the muscle spindle receptors. It seems rather probable
that the findings provided in the present report and
the preceding papers mentioned will apply in principle
also to other neuronal impulse encoders.

METHODS

   Preparation: Adult cats under pentobarbital anaesthesia were spinalized (Th 11/12). The spinal canal was
opened caudal to the third lumbar vertebra, the dura re-
moved and the ventral roots L5 and S1 were sectioned.
The femoral nerve and all nerves of the lower limb except to the M. gastrocnemius lateralis and medialis were
sectioned. The animals were fixed in a special spine
holder. The spinal cord was covered by warm paraffin
oil. The M. gastrocnemius and the M. soleus were prepared and fixed in a heated paraffin pool (36-38°C,fig.1).
A stimulus electrode was fixed around the gastrocnemius
nerve (S1), a second stimulation electrode (S2) was
brought in contact with the proximal ending of the
single primary or secondary afferent fibre. This afferent fiber was prepared from a small filament of the
dorsal root L7 or S1.

   Recording: The action potentials from isolated
primary or secondary afferent fibers were recorded by
means of a silver wire electrode. The bioelectrical
potentials were amplified by a 122 Tectronix preampli-
fier and fed into a Tectronix 565 oscilloscope (2A62
plug-in-unit). The stimulus and the neuronal impulses
were simultaneously tape-recorded (Ampex SP300) and the
average impulse rate was monitored by a Hartmann & Braun
electronic counter.

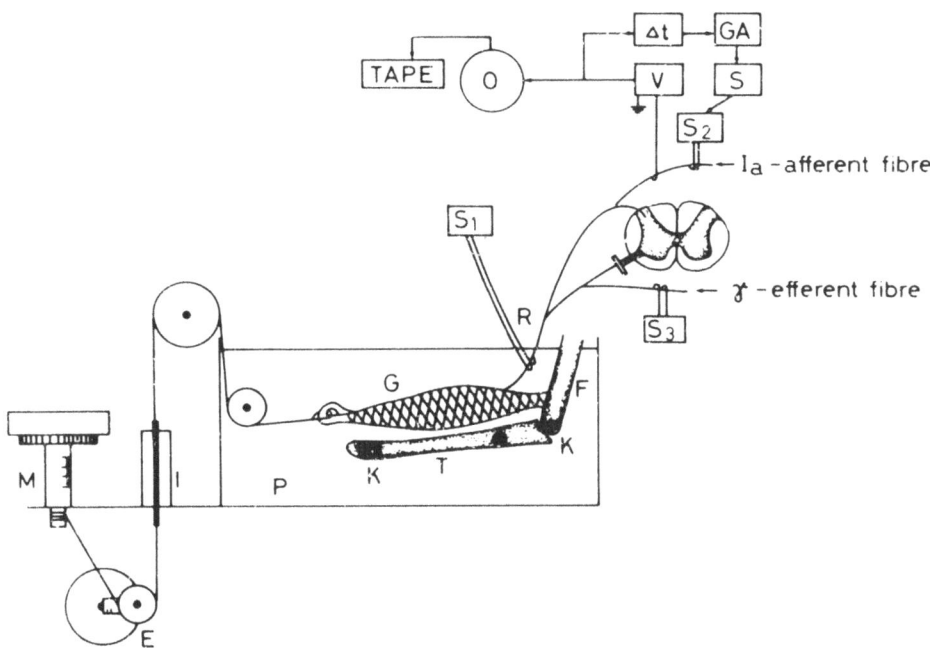

Fig. 1   Schema of the experimental method. G-Gastro-
          cnemius muscle in a heated paraffin pool (P).
          The bones of the leg (T,F) are fixed by a speci-
          al bone holder (K). A stimulus electrode is
          placed around the gastrocnemius nerve (S_1). The
          gastrocnemius muscle can be stretched sinusoid-
          ally or steadily by an excenter (E) or a micro-
          meter screw (M). The length of the muscle is
          measured by an inductive instrument (I). The
          action potentials are recorded from isolated
          afferent fibers, amplified (V) and fed into an
          oscilloscope (O) and into a magnetic tape re-
          corder. The action potential triggers, after
          variable delay Δt an electronic gate, which in
          turn elicits single or repetitive electrical
          stimuli (S) which are used for antidromic sti-
          mulation of the afferent fiber via the trans-
          former S_2. One efferent gamma fiber innervating
          the muscle spindle, from which the recorded af-
          ferent fiber originates, was stimulated via
          stimulus electrode S_3.

     Stimulation: Mechanical stimulation of the gastro-
cnemius muscle and contraction of this muscle by elec-

trical stimulation through stimulus electrode S1 was
applied to prove that the fiber originated from a muscle
spindle of the gastrocnemius muscle. The conduction
velocity of the afferent fiber was calculated from the
latency of the response to stimulation of electrode S1
and the distance between S1 and the recording electrode.

A steady-state, impulse pattern with highly regular
intervals was produced by tonic stretching of the
muscle. The static muscle length could be varied by the
micrometer screw of the stimulus equipment (fig.1). In
some experiments the discharge of the muscle spindle
afferent was increased by additional stimulation of
isolated, efferent, gamma fibers of the static type via
stimulus electrode S3.

Sinusoidal stretch of the gastrocnemius muscle was
applied via the rotating excenter (E) of fig.1. In the
present series of experiments the mechanical stimulus
frequency was restricted to a frequency range below 15
Hz (for details of the mechanical stimulus apparatus
see Grüsser and Thiele, 1968).

The amplified action potentials of the isolated
afferent fiber were fed into a 162 Tectronix pulse
generator. By a variable delay Δt this action potential opened an electronic gate, by which a single
electrical stimulus (0.1   msec duration, 0.8 to 3 volt
amplitude) or a series of electrical stimuli (50-500
stimuli per sec) were applied to the afferent fibers
via stimulus electrode S2 (fig.2). The delay Δt was
variable between 0 and I_b msec, whereby I_b was the impulse interval elicited by the constant stretching. The
duration of a stimulus train and the numbers of stimuli
in a stimulus train were also variable (fig.3 and 4).

Data analysis: All bioelectrical recordings were
taped and later processed by a Linc-8 digital computer.
The programs were written by Mrs. Glathe-Vierkant. The
computer measured single impulse intervals with a precision of 0.2 msec. The consecutive 10 to 50 impulse
intervals after the triggering action potential (fig.2)
were measured, numerated and used for further calculation. 20 to 30 responses for a given Δt were averaged
to obtain the mean values of each impulse interval following the antidromic stimulus. These averaged data
were used for further analysis.

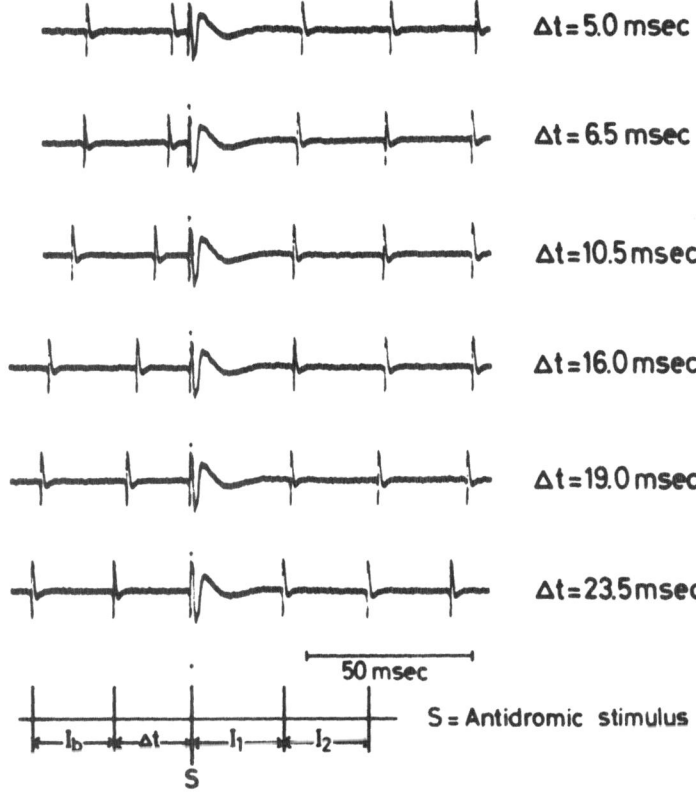

$\Delta t = 5.0$ msec

$\Delta t = 6.5$ msec

$\Delta t = 10.5$ msec

$\Delta t = 16.0$ msec

$\Delta t = 19.0$ msec

$\Delta t = 23.5$ msec

50 msec

S = Antidromic stimulus

I_b — Δt — I_1 — I_2

S

Fig. 2   Recording examples of the impulse pattern of a
         primary afferent fiber (conduction velocity 85
         m.sec^{-1}). Static stretching of the muscle(about
         2 mm above threshold) elicits a regular impulse
         rate with an impulse interval of about 25.5
         msec. By antidromic stimulation, triggered
         after a variable delay Δt by one of the im-
         pulses (stimulus artefact S marked by dots),
         an increase of the next impulse interval (I_1)
         occurs. Increasing delay Δt from top to bottom.

RESULTS

Static Stretch and Antidromic Stimulation

In fig.2, typical responses of an afferent fiber
to antidromic stimulation are shown. By tonic stretching of the gastrocnemius muscle, a very regular impulse
pattern with a mean interval I_b was elicited. As pre-

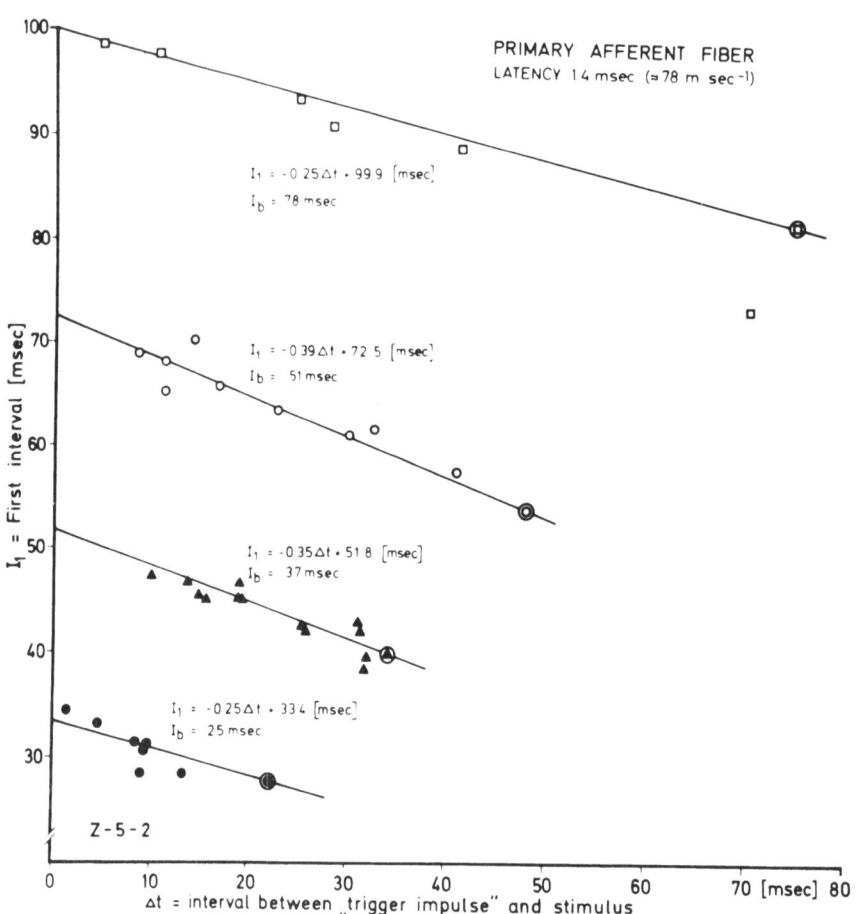

Fig. 3   Relationship between Δt of the antidromic im-
         pulse (abscissa, see fig.2) and the first inter-
         val (I_1) after the antidromic impulse (ordinate).
         Results from a primary afferent fiber (conduc
         tion velocity 78 m.sec^{-1}). The impulse interval
         I_b at the 4 different stretch levels was 67,
         51, 37 and 25 msec. Each symbol represents the
         average of 20 measurements.

dicted by eq. (2), an additional impulse elicited by
antidromic stimulation Δt msec after an orthodromic impulse led to an increase in the next impulse interval
(I_1). The experimental data are well described by the
following linear relation for $t < I_b$ (fig. 3):

$$I_1 = \underline{g}\,\Delta t + k \quad [\text{msec}] \tag{3}$$

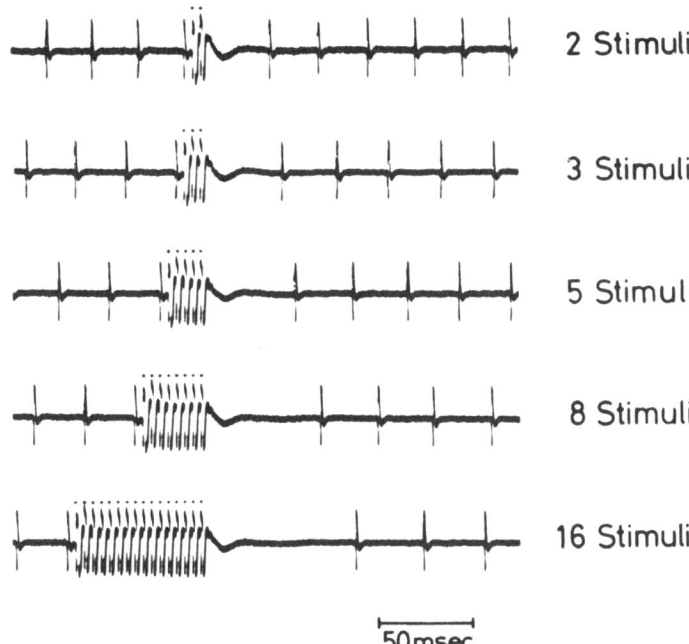

<u>Fig. 4</u>   Impulse pattern of the same primary afferent
         fiber as shown in fig.2. Response to a train of
         antidromic stimuli (Δt = 4.8 msec, stimulus
         frequency - 200 stimuli per sec, impulse inter-
         val before stimulation - 27 msec). The increase
         of the impulse interval I_1 after the end of the
         stimulus train is dependent of the number n_a of
         stimuli in the stimulus train.

The multiplicative constant <u>a</u> in this equation varied
between 0.160 and 0.700, the mean <u>a</u> for 43 units was
0.373 ± 0.019. No correlation between <u>a</u> and the conduction velocity of the afferent fibers was found.

     The impulse frequency on which the antidromic im-
pulses were superimposed was varied by different amounts
of suprathreshold stretch. As fig. 3 shows, the general
validity of eq. (3) was not affected by an increase of
the stretchinduced, impulse frequency from about 10 to
50 impulses.sec^{-1} (100 msec > I_b > 20 msec). Within these
limits the constant of eq. (3) was only slightly influenced by a change of I_b. The absolute value of the
negative multiplicative constant <u>a</u> increased when I_b decreased (I_b < 50 msec, correlation coefficient r = -0.51).

     A train of frequent antidromic impulses increased
the successive impulse interval I_1 more than a single
antidromic stimulus (fig. 4). This result was also expected by eq. (2). In fig. 5 and 6, examples for the

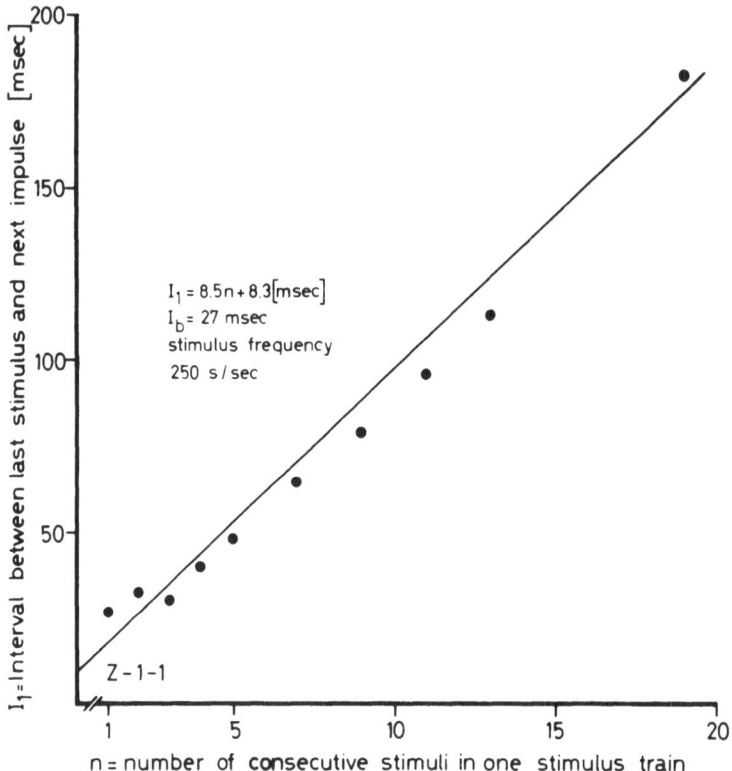

Fig. 5   Relationship between I_1 and the number n_a of
         antidromic stimuli in a stimulus train. Data
         from a primary afferent fiber. Conduction velo-
         city 110 m.sec^{-1}. Frequency of electrical stimuli
         = 250 stimuli per sec. I_b = 27 msec.

quantitative relationship between the first impulse
interval after the antidromic stimulus train and the
numbers of stimuli in a train of constant stimulus
frequencies is shown. With a longer train of frequent
antidromic stimuli, not only the first impulse intervals
after the stimuli but also the successive impulse intervals I_2, I_3 ... increased in duration.

    When less than 20 to 30 stimuli were applied and
the antidromic impulses were elicited at a constant
frequency between 100 and 300 per sec, the relationship
between the number n_a of antidromic impulses and the
length of the first impulse interval I_1 after the antidromic impulse train was approximately a linear function
(fig.5). As fig. 6 demonstrates, this linear relationship
between n_a and I_1 was no longer valid if more than
30 to 50 frequent antidromic impulses were elicited.

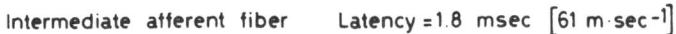

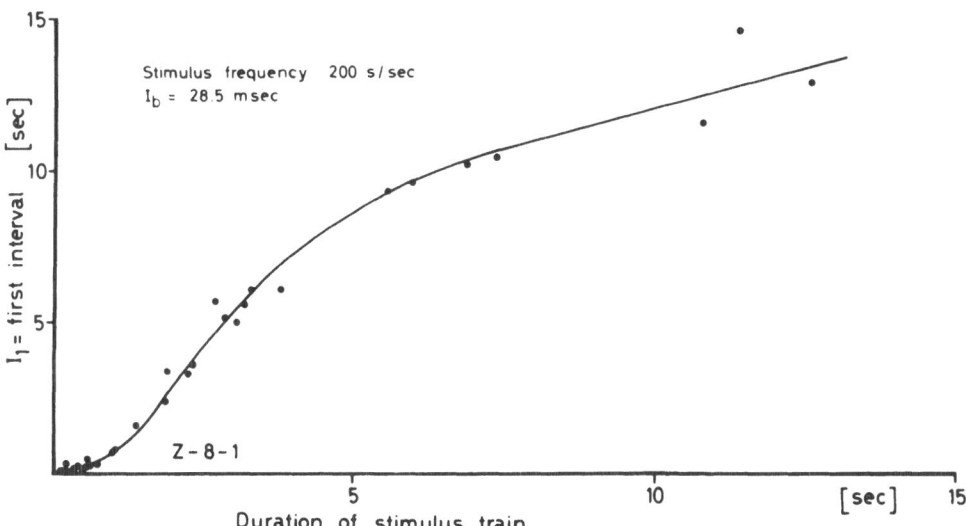

Fig. 6   Dependency of the first interval (I_1 , ordinate,
         see fig. 4) on the duration of the train of the
         antidromic stimuli. Stimulus frequency 200
         stimuli per sec. Results from an intermediate
         afferent fiber, conduction velocity 61 m.sec^{-1} .

Static Stretch, Electrical Stimulation of Static Gamma Efferents and Antidromic Stimulation

     The impulse frequency ($f_b = 1/I_b$) on which the anti-
dromic stimuli were superimposed was varied also by
long-lasting, electrical stimulation of single efferent
gamma fibers isolated from ventral root filaments (80-
150 stimuli per sec). The fluctuation of the impulse
interval I_b was somewhat larger during Gamma-stimulation than without. Therefore, the statistical variability of the experimental data obtained with antidromic
impulses was higher than that of the data described in
section 1. In general, however, the validity of eq. (3)
remained independent of whether I_b was decreased by
gamma-stimulation or by increased static stretch.

Sinusoidal Mechanical Stimulation and
Antidromic Stimulation

In a third series of experiments, the gastrocnemius
muscle was sinusoidally stretched at different frequencies and amplitudes (c.f. Grüsser and Thiele 1968). The
stimuli which elicited additional, antidromically conducted impulses were phase-locked to the sine wave of
the mechanical stimuli, whereby the phase angle ψ between the sinusoidal stimulus and the antidromic impulse
train could be varied arbitrarily. Results from such
experiments are shown in fig.7. When the antidromic impulses were elicited during the pause between the orthodromic impulse group, elicited by the sinusoidal mechanical stimuli, the orthodromic impulse pattern was more
changed, the less the time between antidromic and orthodromic impulses. The latency of the first impulse elicited by each mechanical sine-wave was more increased the
shorter the interval to the preceding antidromic stimulus
train and the higher the number and frequency of the additional antidromic impulses. Fig.7 further shows that
the whole impulse pattern elicited by the mechanical
sine-wave was affected by wellplaced, preceding, antidromic stimuli. Experiments of this type indicate that
due to threshold changes at the encoder side, the receptor potential has to reach higher values in order to
trigger orthodromic impulses. These findings confirm
the opinion of Paintal (1959b), who found with short
mechanical stimuli an increase of the mechanical impulse
threshold after antidromic impulses.

DISCUSSION

Several authors (Henatsch, 1967; Crowe, 1968;
Schäfer and Schäfer, 1969; Rudjord, 1970 a, b; Poppele
and Bowman, 1970) have proposed linear models to describe the relationship between mechanical stimuli and
the responses of muscle spindle afferent fibers. Linear
differential equations of first or second order were
found to be suitable for the description of the input-
output relation of the investigated biological system.
The linear models were derived, as a rule, from the experimental data obtained with positive ramp stretch
(linear increase of the muscle length), but it is easy
to show that the same linear differential equations do
not describe the response with negative ramp stimuli
(linear decrease of the muscle length). Experiments
with sinusoidal stimuli varying in frequency, depth of

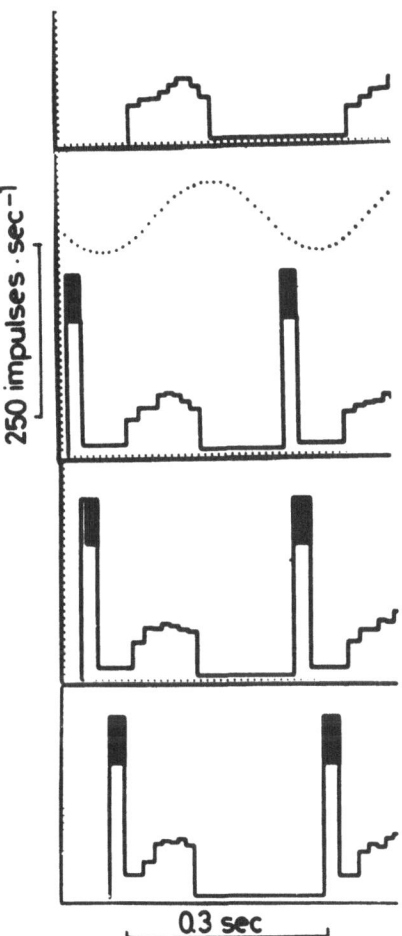

Fig. 7   Impulse pattern of a single primary afferent
         fiber to sinusoidal stretch of the gastrocnemius
         muscle (3Hz,amplitude about 2 mm).The neuronal
         impulse pattern is changed by 7 preceding anti-
         dromic impulses,applied at a frequency of 200
         stimuli per sec.the change of the impulse pat-
         tern elicited by the mechanical stimuli is the
         stronger the shorter the time interval between
         antidromic impulse series and orthodromic im-
         pulse pattern (150,107 and 20 msec).The height
         of the bars represents the instantaneous impulse
         frequency.

modulation, and amplitude revealed that the response of
deefferented muscle spindles of cats can be described
by a linear model only for very small stimulus amplitudes (0.5 mm). Mechanical sine wave amplitudes above
these values lead to non-linear responses of primary
and secondary afferent fibers (Grüsser and Thiele,
1968; Dabbert and Grüsser, 1968; Matthews and Stein,
1969). It was earlier proposed that at least part of
the non-linearity of the muscle spindle response might
be caused by properties of the encoder process (Grüsser
and Thiele, 1968; Eysel and Grüsser, 1970).

The experimental data described in the present report indicate that a temporal summation of the threshold elevations caused by successive impulses at the
encoder (eq. 2) seems to be a useful hypothesis. Eq.(2)
predicts that the non-linearity of the encoder process
becomes apparent if the impulse rate exceeds a certain
minimal frequency and if the modulation of the instantaneous impulse rate is larger than ten to fifteen percent.

For the following considerations let us assume
that the threshold elevations caused by $\underline{n}$ successive impulses are summed. The impulse interval I_b observed at
steady stretch is then:

$$I_b = \frac{k^*}{D} \left(1 + \frac{1}{2} + \frac{1}{3} + \ldots + \frac{1}{n} \right) \tag{4}$$

whereby $D = (MP - \theta_0)$ is the difference between the
receptor's membrane potential MP and the basic thres-
hold θ_0. I_1 can then be calculated as a function of Δt:

$$D = \frac{k^*}{I_1} + \frac{k^*}{I_1 + \Delta t} + \frac{k^*}{I_1 + \Delta t + I_b} + \ldots + \frac{k^*}{I_1 + \Delta t + (n-2)I_b} \tag{5}$$

with $\Delta t = \lambda I_b$ and $I_1 = \xi I_b$ the experimental data are
normalized and the results become independent of I_b.
One obtains from eq. (4) and (5):

$$\sum_{j=1}^{n} \frac{1}{j} = \frac{1}{\xi} + \frac{1}{\xi + \lambda} + \frac{1}{\xi + \lambda + 1} + \ldots + \frac{1}{\xi + \lambda + (n-2)} \tag{6}$$

The experimental data are described well by eq. (6)
when $2 < n < 5$. Of course, the deviation from a linear
relationship between Δt and I_1 as given in eq. (3) increases with larger n. For $n < 5$, however, these deviations are rather small and within the limits of the
statistical variability of our experimental data (fig.8).

   When a train of high frequency antidromic impulses
is elicited (fig. 5,6) it is also possible to use eq.
(2) for the prediction of the experimental data. When
n in eq. (2) is restricted to 6 and $\alpha(t) = 0$, the experimental data are fitted very well, as long as the
number of antidromic impulses does not exceed 20 to 30.
Under these conditions there is an approximately linear
relationship between I_1 and the number of antidromic
stimuli n_a. When the number of antidromically conducted
impulses in a stimulus train exceeds 20 to 30, eq. (2)
no longer predicts the experimental data (fig. 6). We
assume that by such long lasting high frequency discharges not only the encoder site but also the receptor
site of the muscle spindle afferents is affected.

   Eq. (2) can be also applied to explain the change
of the impulse pattern elicited by mechanical stimuli
by means of preceding, antidromic, impulse trains. A
complete simulation of the experimental data presented
in the present report will be described in another paper
(Eysel and Grüsser,1973).

   Our experimental and theoretical results indicate,
that for a complete description of the input-output
function of a muscle spindle's receptive mechanisms the
non-linear properties of the encoder have to be considered. The impulse encoder acts as a linear device
only under very restricted conditions. Hence, the application of linear differential equations to the description of this receptor's function is a very restricted one. Also, within intact gamma innervation, a great
part of the muscle spindle's physiological working
range falls far beyond the validity of linear models.
Comparative studies of the responses of motoneurones'
primary, afferent input and of the output impulse pattern of alpha motoneurones indicate that at the side
of the motoneuron, another non-linear transformation
counteracts the receptor's non-linearity. Therefore the
overall feedback mechanism of muscle, muscle spindles
and spinal cord might act as a whole more like a linear
system than its single parts.

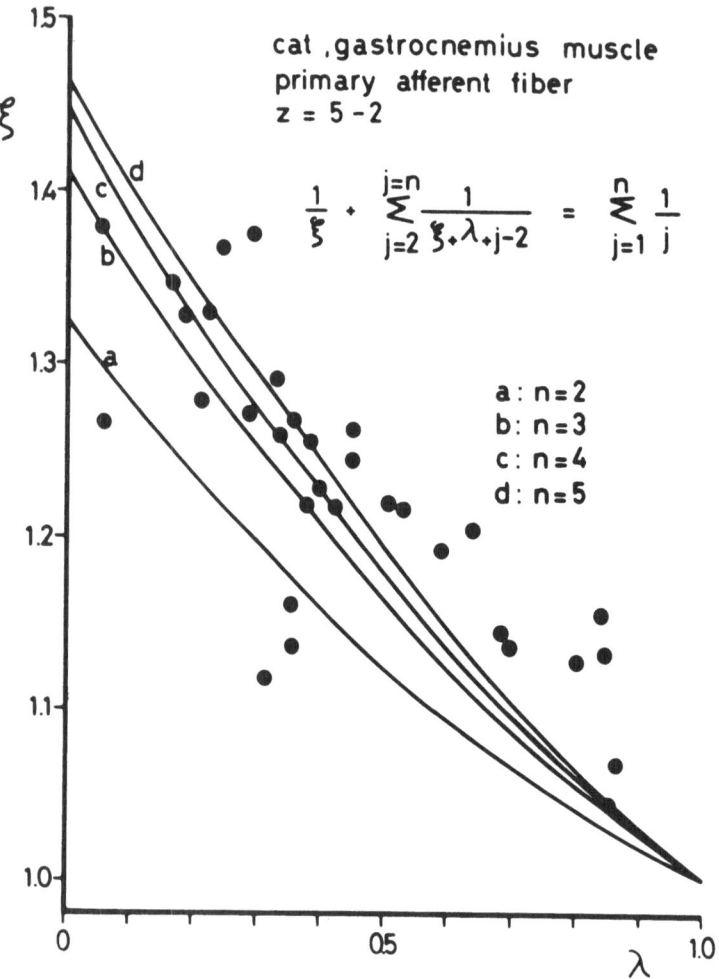

$$\frac{1}{\xi} + \sum_{j=2}^{j=n} \frac{1}{\xi + \lambda + j - 2} = \sum_{j=1}^{n} \frac{1}{j}$$

<u>Fig. 8</u> Data of fig. 3 in normalized presentation. The
delay Δt is given on the abscissa as fraction
λ of I_b. On the ordinate I_1 is given as fraction
ξ of I_b. The curves are calculated from eq. (6),
when the temporal summation of threshold elevation is restricted to 2, 3, 4 and 5 preceding
impulses.

SUMMARY

It was earlier proposed that the transformation of
the receptor potential into impulse sequences in mammalian muscle spindle afferents (encoder process) could
be characterized by the change of the threshold after

an impulse and, in addition, by a limited temporal summation of the threshold elevations which remain after
each impulse of a fast sequence of impulses. These properties of the encoder process would explain the sequential dependence found for the impulse pattern of muscle
spindle afferents. Some non-linear properties of the
signal transfer, found when mechanical stimuli are applied to the muscle, are also predictable by these encoder properties.

The present report deals with properties of this
encoder process. The experiments were performed in
primary and secondary afferent fibers from the gastrocnemius muscle of the cat.

The hypothesis of temporal summation of threshold
elevation was tested directly by the application of antidromically elicited action potentials. The antidromic
impulses were added to the impulse sequence elicited by
steady stretch of the muscle or by sinusoidal mechanical
stimuli. The antidromic impulses were triggered with a
variable delay Δt by the orthodromic action potentials
of the afferent fibers. The number and the frequency of
antidromic impulses elicited by a stimulus train were
also variable. The change of the impulse pattern caused
by the antidromic stimuli was quantitatively analysed.
The results support the hypothesis that above a certain
impulse frequency and above a change of the impulse rate
of ten to fifteen percent, the encoder acts as a non-
linear device for the transformation of the receptor
potential into an impulse sequence. The data are
quantitatively described by a simple mathematical model.
In this model the change of the threshold is described
by the sum of a limited number of hyperbolic time functions.

REFERENCES

CROWE, A. (1968). A mechanical model of the mammalian
   muscle spindle. J.Theor.Biol. 21: 21-41
DABBERT, H., GRÜSSER, O.-J. (1968). Reaktionen primärer
   und sekundärer Muskelspindelafferenzen auf sinus-
   förmige mechanische Reizung. II. Änderung der stati-
   schen Vordehnung. Pflügers Arch.Physiol. 304: 258-270.
EYSEL, U.Th. (1971). Computer simulation of the impulse pattern of muscle spindle afferents under static
   and dynamic conditions. Kybernetik 8: 171-179
EYSEL, U.Th., GRÜSSER, O.-J. (1970). The impulse pattern of muscle spindle afferents - A statistical ana-

lysis of the response to static and sinusoidal stimulation. Pflügers Arch. Physiol. 315: 1-26

EYSEL, U.Th., GRÜSSER, O.-J. (1973). The change of the
impulse pattern of muscle spindle afferents by antidromic impulses. Kybernetik (in press)

GRÜSSER, O.-J., THIELE, B. (1968). Reaktionen primärer
und sekundärer Muskelspindelafferenzen auf sinusför-
mige mechanische Reizung. I. Variation der Sinusfre-
quenz. Pflügers Arch.Physiol. 300: 161-184.

HENATSCH, H.D. (1967). Instability of the proprioceptive length servo: Its possible role in tremor phenomena. In: Neurophysiological basis of normal and abnormal motor activities. Proceedings of the 3rd Symposium of Parkinsons' disease, ed. M.D. Yahr and D.P.
Purpura, p.75-90. Hewlett: Raven press

MATTHEWS, B.H.C. (1931). The response of a muscle spindle
during active contraction of a muscle. J.Physiol.
(Lond.) 72: 153-174

MATTHEWS, B.H.C. (1933). Nerve endings in mammalian
muscle. J.Physiol.(Lond.) 78: 1-53

MATTHEWS, P.B.C. (1964). Muscle spindles and their
motor control. Physiol.Rev. 44: 219-288

MATTHEWS, P.B.C., STEIN, R.B. (1969). The sensitivity
of muscle spindle afferents to small sinusoidal
changes of length. J.Physiol.(Lond.) 200: 723-743

PAINTAL, A.S. (1959a). Intramuscular propagation of
sensory impulses. J.Physiol. (Lond.) 148: 240-251

PAINTAL, A.S. (1959b). Facilitation and depression of
muscle stretch receptors by repetitive antidromic
stimulation, adrenaline, and asphyxia. J.Physiol.
(Lond.) 148: 252-266.

POPPELE, R.E., BOWMAN, R.J. (1970). Quantitative description of linear behavior of mammalian muscle
spindles. J.Neurophysiol. 33: 59-72

RUDJORD, T. (1970a). A second order mechanical model of
muscle spindle primary endings. Kybernetik 6: 205-
213

RUDJORD, T. (1970b). A mechanical model of the secondary
endings of mammalian spindles. Kybernetik 7: 122-128

SCHÄFER, S.S., SCHÄFER, S. (1968). Die Eigenschaften
einer primären Muskelspindelafferenz bei rampenförmi-
ger Dehnung und ihre mathematische Beschreibung.
Pflügers Arch.Physiol. 310: 206-228

IMPULSE ACTIVITY FROM HUMAN MUSCLE SPINDLES DURING VOLUNTARY CONTRACTIONS

Å. B. VALLBO

From the Department of Physiology, Biological
Institute, University of Umeå
Sweden

The present report gives a summary of the main findings obtained in analysis of the impulse discharge in
single muscle spindle afferents in conscious human subjects. The results have been published in earlier papers
which may be consulted for further information (Vallbo,
1970 a,b, 1971, 1972 a,b).

The recording method was developed in 1964 and it
was continuously refined in the following few years
(Vallbo and Hagbarth, 1968). In short the method implies
that fine needle electrodes are inserted percutaneously
towards a limb nerve, one of them right into the nerve.
The exact position of the recording electrode is then
adjusted in very small steps until the type of activity
of interest is recorded.

The electrodes are tungsten needles pointed electro-
lytically to a tip diameter of about ten microns, they
are insulated with Araldite (type AZ 15, CIBA) to about
30 microns from the very tip, which has a diameter of
5-15 microns. This gives an impedance of around 1 kohm
at 1 kHz.

The electrodes are inserted through the skin and
the tissues as they are without any particular arrangements for protecting the tip. Usually the tip takes the
mechanical strain reasonably well but not too seldom it
may be damaged when the electrode passes through very
tough tissues. All through the experiment the electrodes
are manipulated with a rather ordinary pair of forceps

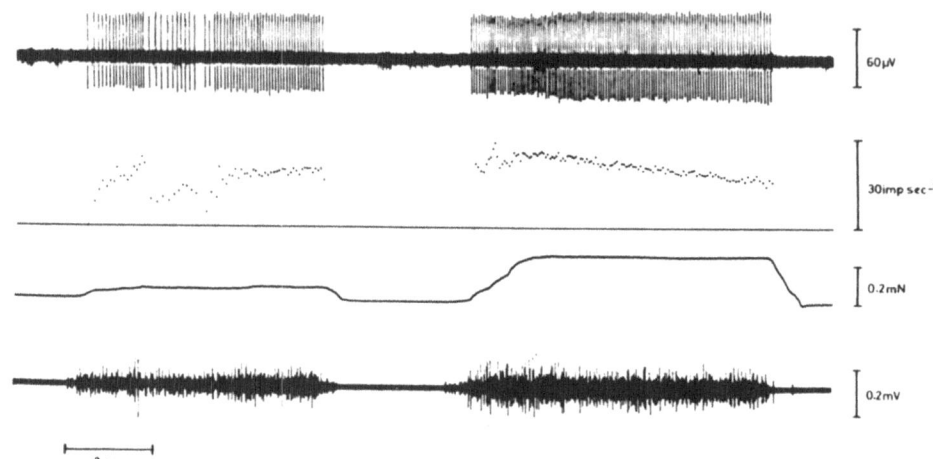

60 µV

30 imp sec⁻¹

0.2 mN

0.2 mV

2 sec

Fig. 1   Afferent unitary discharge associated with two
         successive voluntary contractions, without ex-
         ternal shortening, of the flexor muscles acting
         on the index. From above are shown the unitary
         nerve impulses, the instantaneous impulse fre-
         quency, the torque due to contraction and the
         electromyographic activity recorded with surface
         electrodes. The straight line indicates zero im-
         pulse frequency. The torque is given in metre-
         newton (mN). (Vallbo, 1970a, Acta physiol.Scand.)

and they are left freely floating in the tissues.

     The data to be presented were all obtained in re-
cordings from the median nerve on the upper arm and the
endings were all located in the long finger flexor
muscles which have their muscle bellies on the forearm.

     When you ask the subject to contract the muscle in
which the spindle you are recording from is located, the
spindle discharge increases as shown in Fig. 1. The two
contractions in this figure were done under isometric
conditions. The mechanical effects of the contraction on
the muscle spindle would be to unload it to some extent.
However, the discharge actually increased and this indicates that the fusimotor activity actually increases
and well compensates for the unloading effect. This type
of response was found in the vast majority of the spindles, providing the subject activated the muscle in which
the spindle was located (Vallbo,1970 b). This finding
indicates that the fusimotor system is strongly engaged
in voluntary contractions in man and that the fusimotor
outflow during voluntary contraction is largely restricted to the contracting muscle.

    In animal experiments it has been found that the
fusimotor activity and the spindle afferent discharge
precedes the muscle contraction when a motor act is initiated (for ref. see Granit, 1970). This has been found
in electrical stimulation of central structures and in a
number of reflexes. The finding has been taken as a
support for the idea that muscles are largely controlled
indirectly through the muscle spindle reflex loop. In
its extreme form, this is the follow-up length servo
hypothesis (Merton, 1951). However, it will be shown that
in voluntary contractions in man this hypothesis must be
rejected. The findings to be presented on this point are
specifically concerned with the following questions. Is
it possible to reveal any clear principle with regard to
the relative time of onset of the activity in the skeletomotor and the fusimotor system? Does one regularly start
before the other or does it vary from one test to the
other? And if it does vary, is it possible to find the
determining factors or are the respective onsets unpredictable?

    The time of onset of spindle acceleration was de-
termined in relation to the time of onset of the electromyographic activity in the appropriate muscles. The subject performed on instruction, isometric contractions.
In the vast majority of tests that was flexion of one
particular finger. Figure 2 shows the basic findings.
The top record of each pair shows the impulses from a
muscle spindle primary ending, the second one is the
electromyographic activity. The subject repeated the
same contraction four times. It is seen, that the activity in the skeletomotor system regularly precedes the
onset of the spindle acceleration and that there is no
constant time lag between the two activities. This was
valid both for slowly rising contractions and for rapidly rising contractions, as shown in Fig. 3 B and C. The
small isometric muscle twitches are associated with
bursts of impulses from the spindle and these appear
clearly after the onset of the skeletomotor contractions.
Incidentally, the records in A show that unloading effects may be obtained, in this particular case, when the
contractions were somewhat more slowly rising.

    If you ask the subject to repeat the same contrac-
tion over and over again you may collect a sample of
observations concerning the time lag between the onset
of the activity in the two systems. Figure 4 shows three
samples from three different units. The histograms give
the time lag between the two events. Values to the right

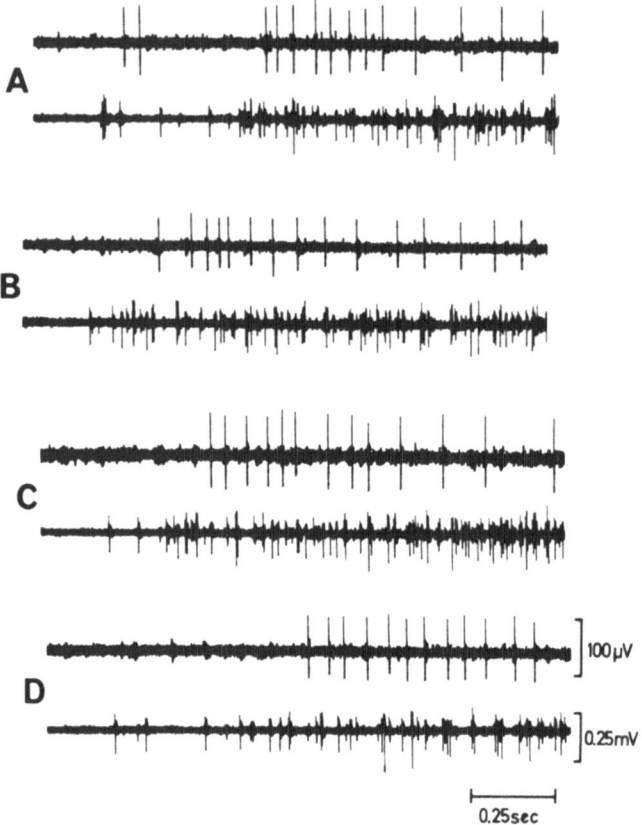

Fig. 2   Discharges from a single muscle spindle ending
         (upper traces)and the electromyographic activity
         of the long finger flexor muscles (lower traces)
         associated with the onset of isometric voluntary
         flexions of the ring finger, The electromyograph-
         ic activity was recorded with a needle electrode
         inserted in close vicinity of the receptor which
         was located 7 cm distally to the elbow. (From
         Vallbo, 1971, J.Physiol. London).

of zero indicate that spindle acceleration lags the
onset of the skeletomotor activity. It may be seen that
in practically all the tests, spindle acceleration lags
after the onset of the skeletomotor activity. The same
was found in the rest of the samples for slowly rising
as well as for rapidly rising contractions. From this
finding it may be concluded, first that the fusimotor
system is not involved in the initiation of voluntary
contractions, but the start of a voluntary contraction
must be the consequence of descending impulses from
supraspinal structures and their influence upon the
segmental organization within the spinal cord, most

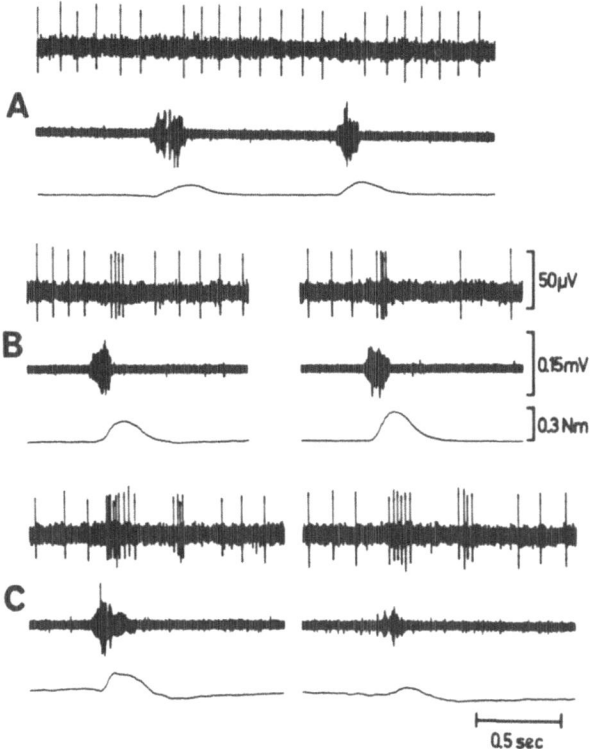

Fig. 3   Afferent discharge from a single muscle spindle
          ending (upper traces), electromyographic activ-
          ity (middle traces) and torque due to active
          contraction (lower traces) during isometric
          flexions of the ring finger. The electromyograph-
          ic activity was recorded with a needle electrode
          inserted in the vicinity of the receptor.(From
          Vallbo, 1971, J. Physiol. London).

probably through direct effects upon the alfa motoneurones. Second, it may be concluded, that the voluntary
contractions are not totally servo controlled through
the muscle spindle reflex loop- as the initial part
clearly is not. Thus the follow-up length servo hypothesis must be rejected for these types of contractions
(Vallbo,1971).

    However, it may be argued that the initial part of
a contraction is a rather particular process which might
be controlled in another way than the rest of a contraction, and it may be maintained that a sustained contraction is largely controlled according to the servo hypothesis - except for the very initial part. The findings

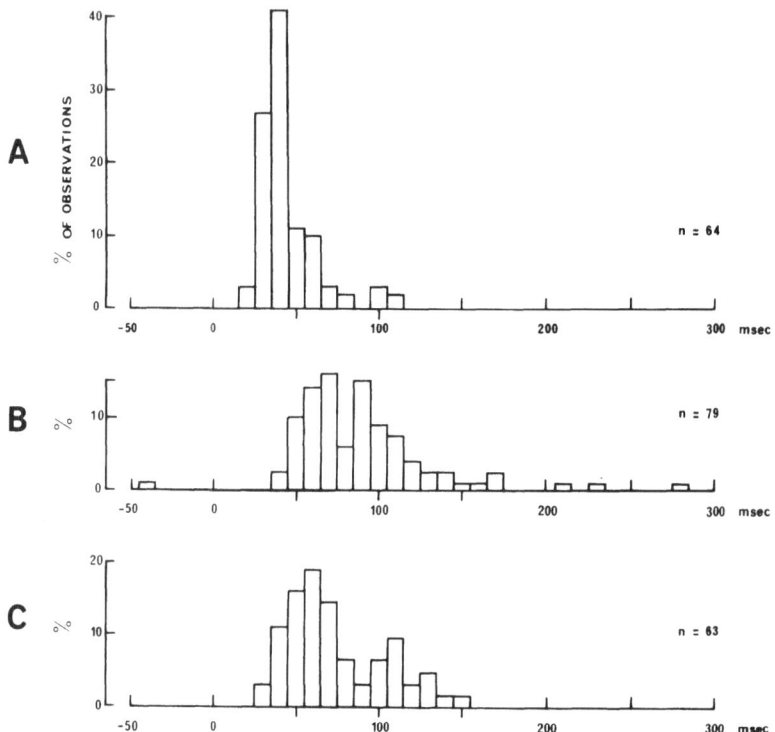

Fig. 4   Histograms showing the distribution of time lags
         between the onset of the skeletomotor activity,
         as determined from the electromyographic activ‐
         ity, and the onset of spindle acceleration when
         the subject performed isometric twitches. Find‐
         ings from three spindle endings are shown in A,
         B and C respectively. (From Vallbo, 1971, J.
         Physiol. London).

to be presented below indicate that this is not the
case.

     According to the follow-up length servo hypothesis
the intensity of the skeletomotor output would be
closely related to the intensity of the muscle spindle
afferent inflow since this inflow is what is driving
the skeletomotor neurones. This would be so in isometric
as well as in isotonic contractions. On the other hand,
if it were found that the spindle responds very clearly
to the muscle length and the rate of change of the
muscle length, this would be an argument against the
follow-up length servo hypothesis.

     A few examples of isotonic contractions which are
considered representative, are shown in Figs.5 and 6.

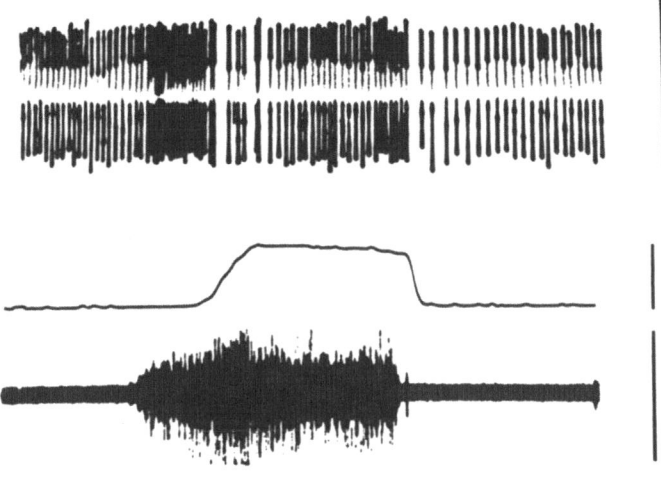

Fig. 5   Response from a spindle primary ending to an
         isotonic contraction. From top to bottom are
         shown the single unit impulses, the angle at
         the metacarpo-phalangeal joint and the
         electromyographic activity when the subject
         flexed his ring finger. The flexion was opposed
         by a load corresponding to a torque of 0.1 mN
         at the metacarpo-phalangeal joint. Calibrations:
         100 μV, 150° (bottom) and 140° (top), 0.2 mV.
         Time signal: 1.0 sec. (From Vallbo, 1972 b, New
         Developments in Electromyography and Clinical
         Neurophysiology, Karger)

In Fig. 5 are seen from above, the muscle spindle impulses, the angle at the metacarpo-phalangeal joint and
the electromyographic activity when the subject flexes
one of his fingers against a small load. If the impulse
frequency is compared with the electromyographic activity, it is obvious that these two variables do not follow each other very well. On the other hand, comparing
the spindle discharge rate with the signal of the joint
angle, it may be seen that initially, when the muscle
is longer the spindle frequency is high, whereas, it is
much lower, as the muscle shortens. During the actual
shortening the impulse frequency is still lower. Thus,
it seems that this spindle discharge is partly a function of an increased fusimotor activity, partly of the
muscle length and the rate of change of the muscle
length during the isotonic contraction.

    Another example is shown in Fig. 6. Here the upper

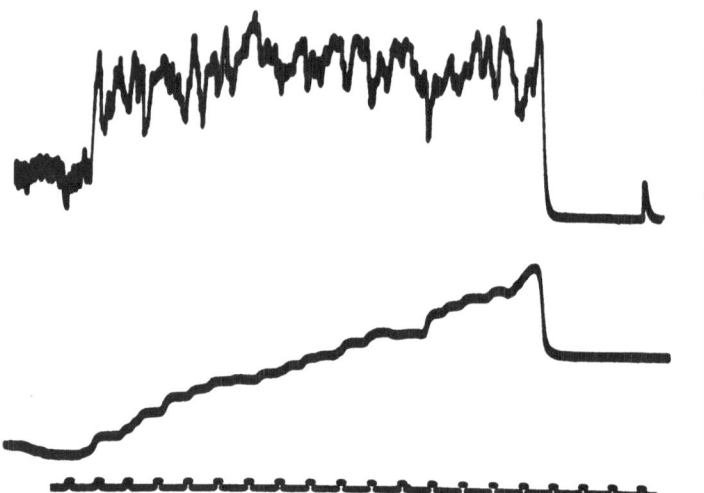

Fig. 6   Response of a muscle spindle primary ending
         during an isotonic contraction. The top trace
         represents the impulse frequency of the single
         unit and the lower trace the angle at the meta-
         carpo-phalangeal joint when the subject slowly
         flexed his ring finger. Calibrations: 0 and 25
         impulses/sec., 155° (bottom) and 145° (top).
         Time signal: 1.0 sec. (From Vallbo, 1972 b, New
         Developments in Electromyography and Clinical
         Neurophysiology, Karger).

signal shows in an analog form the discharge frequency
from a single spindle during an isotonic contraction,
whereas the lower signal represents the angle at the
metacarpo-phalangeal joint while the subject is slowly
flexing his finger. As soon as the contraction starts,
the spindle discharge increases considerably and re-
mains high during the whole movement. Although it varies
a lot up and down, there is not much of a systematic
change of the frequency which could be related to the
continuous muscle shortening. So in this test it seems
as if the muscle spindle was relatively insensitive to
the muscle length. However, an alternative interpretation is that there is a continuous increase of the fusimotor outflow which compensates for the muscle shortening, so that the net result would be spindle discharge
which does not change appreciably as a function of the
muscle length. Considering the small and fast changes
of the impulse frequency as seen in the top record of
Fig. 6 it may be asked whether these are in any way related to the changes of the muscle length. It is obvious that, at least, at one point when the movement

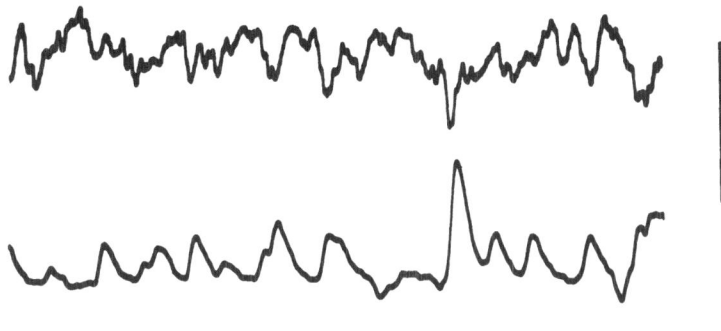

<u>Fig. 7</u>   Response of a muscle spindle primary ending
           during an isotonic contraction related to the
           speed of joint movement. Same events as in
           Fig. 6. The upper trace shows the single unit
           impulse frequency and the lower trace shows the
           time derivative of the joint angle signal or
           the speed of the joint movement. Calibrations:
           0 and 25 impulses/sec. Time signal: 1.0 sec.
           (From Vallbo, 1972 b, New Developments in
           Electromyography and Clinical Neurophysiology,
           Karger).

progresses a little faster, there is a pronounced drop in
the impulse frequency. This indicates that the spindle
might respond to the velocity of movement, if not to the
muscle length itself.

        In order to have a closer look at the relation be-
tween the speed of joint movement and the spindle discharge rate, it would be convenient to have the time
derivative of the joint angle signal. Figure 7 shows a
section of the same events as in Fig. 6 on an expanded
time scale, but now the bottom record is the time
derivative of the joint angle signal, i.e. an approxima-
tion of the speed of muscle shortening during the isotonic contraction, whereas the upper record represents
the discharge rate of the spindle. It may be seen that
these two signals go in opposite directions during the
major part of this sequence, implying that the faster
the muscle is shortening, the lower is the discharge
rate of the spindle and vice versa.

        The implication of this finding is that the ex-
citatory drive onto the skeletomotor neurones through
the muscle spindle reflex loop decreases immediately if
the movement progresses faster, and the excitatory

drive increases if the movement progresses slower. In
this way, any variations in the speed of movement would
be reduced in amplitude and the result would be a smooth-
er movement - and that is regardless of whether these
variations are induced by variations in the load on the
muscle, variations in the frictional resistance of variations in the excitatory drive onto the skeletomotor neurones from other sources. On the other hand, considering
the follow-up length servo hypothesis, you would rather
expect the opposite finding in this type of experiment,
that is that the two signals would follow each other in
the ups and downs.

In summary it may be concluded that the follow-up
length servo hypothesis should be rejected in voluntary
contractions of this type; the muscle contractions are
clearly controlled by means of a combined excitation of
the fusimotor and the skeletomotor neurones from supraspinal structures, i.e. an alfa-gamma linkage. However,
the onset of the contraction is obviously controlled
through the alpha motoneurones alone.The findings present further arguments that one of the functions of the
fusimotor system and the muscle spindles would be to
eliminate variations in the speed of movement and thus
to make the movement progress smoothly and fluently.

REFERENCES

GRANIT, R. (1970). The basis of motor control. London,
  New York: Academic Press.
MERTON, P. A. (1951). The silent period in a muscle of
  the human hand. J..Physiol.(Lond.) 114: 183-198.
VALLBO, Å. B. (1970 a). Slowly adapting muscle receptors
  in man. Acta physiol. scand. 78: 315-333.
VALLBO, Å. B. (1970 b). Discharge patterns in human
  muscle spindle afferents during isometric voluntary
  contractions. Acta physiol. scand. 80: 552-566.
VALLBO, Å. B. (1971). Muscle spindle response at the
  onset of isometric voluntary contractions in man.
  Time difference between fusimotor and skeletomotor
  effects. J.Physiol.(Lond.) 218: 405-431.
VALLBO, Å. B. (1972 a). Single unit recording from
  human peripheral nerves: muscle receptor discharge in
  resting muscles and during voluntary contractions.
  In: "Neurophysiology studied in Man", ed. G. G. Somjen,
  pp. 281-295. Amsterdam:Excerpta Medica.

VALLBO, Å. B. (1972 b). Muscle spindle afferent dis-
    charge from resting and contracting muscles in normal
    subjects. In "New Developments in Electromyography and
    Clinical Neurophysiology", ed. J. E. Desmedt, vol.3,
    pp. 317-324. Basel: Karger.
VALLBO, Å. B. and HAGBARTH, K.-E. (1968). Activity from
    skin mechanoreceptors recorded percutaneously in awake
    human subjects. Expl.Neurol. 21: 270-289.

IMPULSE DECODING PROCESS IN STRETCH REFLEX

S.HOMMA and K.KANDA

From the Department of Physiology, School of
Medicine

Chiba University
Chiba, Japan

Forced vibration of muscle gives rise to a very
gradually increasing tonic contraction which has been
called tonic vibration reflex, TVR (Hagbarth and Eklund,
1966 a, b). Detailed observation of EMG spikes during
TVR revealed that the neuro-motor units mostly fired at
intervals which corresponded to the integer multiples of
the cyclic time of the vibration applied and that the
integer decreased as TVR augmented (Homma, Kanda and
Watanabe, 1971a). It has been firmly established that
muscular Ia afferents precisely correspond to the
vibratory cycle provided the amplitude of vibration applied to the muscle is enough to excite the terminals
at their maximum efficiency (Kuffler, Hunt and Quilliam,
1951; Granit and Henatsch, 1956). In a series of previous papers it was investigated that such afferent spikes
as above are transmitted to the motoneurone which de-
codes them into a slower rate of efferent impulses by
the reciprocals of several arbitrary integers, the diminution ratio being proposed as "decoding ratio" (Homma,
Kanda and Watanabe, 1972). It was also known that condition of α - rigidity provoked lesser decoding ratios and
that this was also observed when facilitation was effected upon the motoneuronal membrane either through
reciprocal or proprioceptive neuronal circuits. It was
suggested that the gradual increment of muscular contraction during vibration was effected by a gradually increasing facilitatory influence activated through some

specific neuronal circuits within the spinal cord. The
present report deals with further investigation of the
activity of such polysynaptic circuits which might play
a very important role when the motoneurone receives a
sustained impingement of Ia impulses due to vibration
of human, monkey and cat muscles.

METHOD

Unitary EMG spikes were recorded at Mm.quadriceps
femoris and triceps surae in human and monkey experiments through bipolar Teflon-insulated copper wire of
80 μ diameter inserted into muscles. Monkeys were an-
esthetized by a 10 - 15 mg/Kg injection of Ketanine
(Ketalar,Sankyo Co., Tokyo) and were fixed in a monkey
apparatus in sitting position. The awakening phase
from anesthesia was found most adequate as the experimental condition for the observation of TVR. No anaesthesia was performed in the human experiment. In the
cat experiment both a decerebrate preparation by suck-
ing and the intact C.N.S. preparation under moderate
chloralose-urethane anaesthesia were used. Mm.gastro-
cnemius and soleus were carefully separated and the
tendon of each muscle was cut and isolated for application of independent longitudinal sinusoidal stretch.
Motoneuronal activity at L7 - S1 segments were recorded
intracellulary by 3M-KCl glass microelectrodes. Simultaneous EMG and stretch activities were monitored in
every experiment. Technical detail of muscle vibration
and data processing has been previously published (Homma,
Ishikawa and Stuart, 1970; Homma et al., 1972).

RESULTS

1. Decoding Ratio in Man, Monkey and Cat

EMG spike activities were recorded in M.quadriceps
femoris in the human experiments and in M.triceps surae
in the monkey and cat experiments, where vibratory
stimulation was applied at their tendons. In Fig. 1A are
shown records of two typical time courses of the reflex
contraction which appeared when human and monkey muscles
received vibratory stimulation. As seen in the figure
the human TVR shows a steady increment while in the
monkey there is an abrupt increase and then gradual decrease of the tension (Homma, Kanda and Watanabe, 1971b).

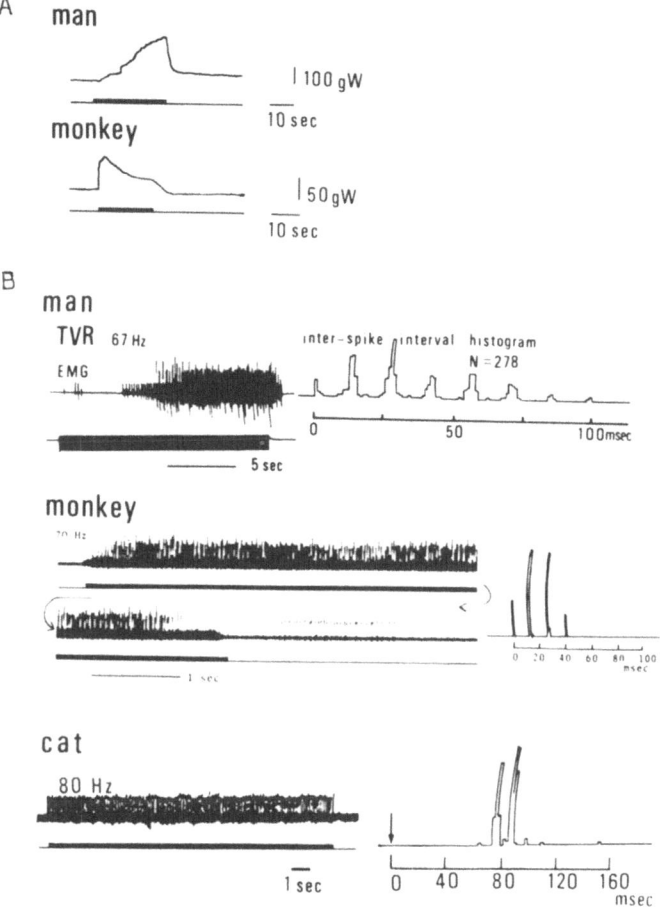

<u>Fig. 1</u>   Tonic vibration reflexes in human, monkey and
          cat muscles. A shows reflex contractions of the
          human quadriceps femoris and monkey triceps
          surae, B shows human quadriceps femoris, monkey
          triceps surae and cat triceps surae muscles dur-
          ing muscle vibration and their corresponding
          inter-spike interval histograms. Each histogram
          displays several peaks separated by the same
          interval which coincide with the cyclic time of
          the vibration applied

     In Fig. 1B are shown unitary EMG activities during
vibration which were recorded in the human, monkey and
cat muscles. To the right of EMG recordings are shown
corresponding inter-spike interval histograms. As clearly seen in the figure each histogram displays several
peaks separated by one and the same time - interval

which coincides with the cyclic time of the vibration
applied (15 ms). This fundamental finding can be generalized as follows: every motor unit fires at intervals
corresponding to some unpredictable multiples of the
cyclic time of the vibration applied. This notion has
been maintained in our preceding reports and was proposed as "principle of integer multiplication", the value
of the integer reciprocal being the decoding ratio mentioned above (Homma et al., 1971a).

2. Muscular Afferent Discharges during Muscle
Vibration in the Cat

Unitary muscle afferents were recorded at L7 - S1
dorsal root filaments of cats under moderate anaesthesia
with urethane-chloralose. Routine criteria were employed
to identify Ia, II and Ib fibers. Fig. 2 shows typical
examples of Ia, II and Ib fiber activities during vibration with intensities at which a one to one correspondence between afferent impulses and vibration was attained.

It is noticed in Figure 2 that the vibratory intensities needed for the full excitation of II and Ib
endings were much higher than that for Ia (Bessou and
Laporte, 1962; Bianconi and Van der Meulen, 1963; Brown,
Engberg and Matthews, 1967). Though not shown in the
figure, Ia endings were in general sensitive for vibratory stimulation between 30 and 200 Hz (Grüsser and Tie-
le, 1968; Fukuda, 1972).

Around 100 Hz a small excursion was enough to
elicit good driving of Ia endings but in most cases
the same amplitude failed to excite both II and Ib endings.

It can be therefore supposed that most of the TVRs
observed at the small amplitudes of vibration are closely associated with excitation of Ia afferents only
(Bianconi and Van der Meulen, 1963; Crowe and Matthews,
1964; Brown et al., 1967).

3. EPSPs Produced by Ia Impulses during Vibration

For further detailed observation of motoneuronal
activity during TVR it seemed essential to investigate
at cellular level how Ia afferents are driving moto-

50 Hz VIBRATION

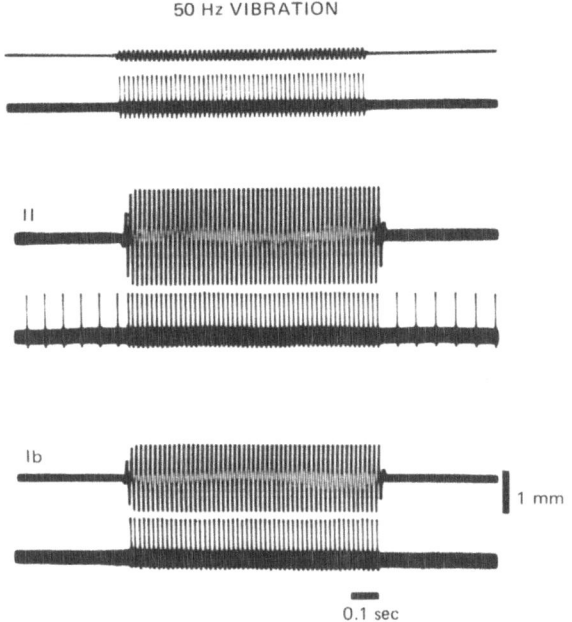

Fig. 2   Unitary muscle afferent discharges at L7 dorsal
         root filaments in the cat. Each upper curve
         shows the minimum amplitude of a vibration of
         50 Hz for full excitation of Ia, II and Ib fibers
         which are shown in the lower traces(Fukuda,1972).

neuronal firing. Cat gastrocnemius motoneurones of L7 –
S1 segments were therefore penetrated by micropipette
electrode in order to record EPSPs and intermittent
firing during muscle vibration of 100 Hz. Typical examples of records from this experiment are shown in
Fig. 3C – F.

   Close correspondence between EPSP ripples and 100
Hz vibration could be invariably noticed even when
vibratory intensities were varied at four steps from C
to F: 48, 94, 144 and 240 μ respectively. It is also
noticed in the records C – F that larger vibratory excursions generate EPSPs with larger amplitude. This
relationship can be explained if the number of Ia impulses which converge to the gastrocnemius motoneurone
gradually increases and this might be the very case
when the vibratory intensity is increased gradually.

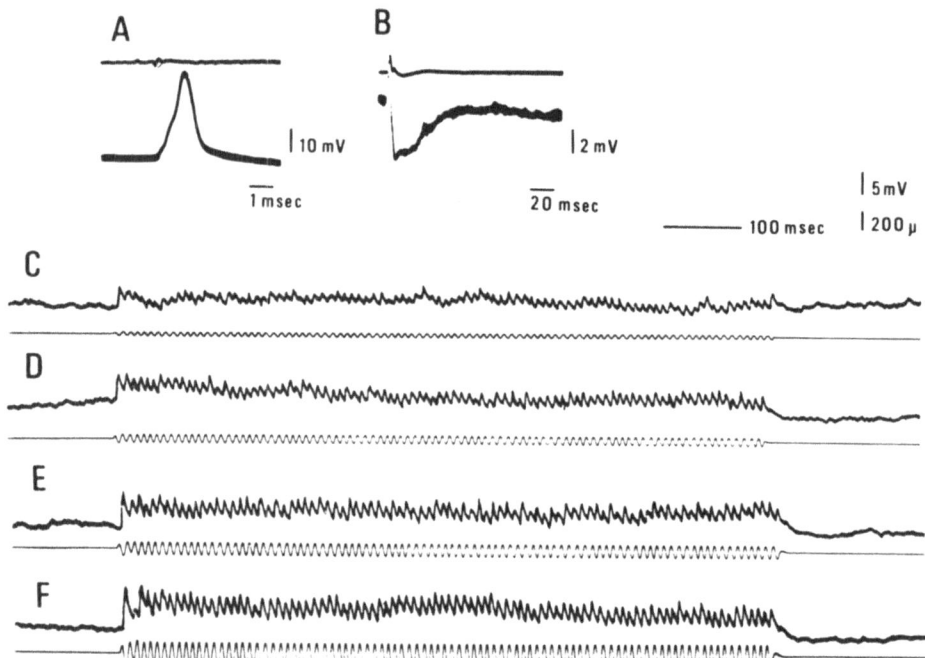

Fig. 3 Cat gastrocnemius motoneurone. A and B show
        orthodromic and antidromic responses respective-
        ly. Each upper trace shows mass potentials re-
        corded by electrode leads at the entrance of the
        dorsal root into the spinal cord. Records from
        C to F show EPSP ripples during 100 Hz vibra-
        tion when the vibratory intensities are varied
        at four steps. Larger vibratory excursions
        generate larger EPSPs.

Another fact which can be noticed in Fig. 3 is a parallel d.c. shift of the motoneuronal membrane potential
towards depolarization as the vibratory stimulation increases. Such sustained depolarization as observed during vibration might well play a facilitatory role in the
firing of the motoneurone involved in TVR. It is also
noticed at the end of the vibratory stimulation (in C -
F) that the membrane potential is recovered with a
relatively slow decay. It has been generally noticed
that the falling phase of this sustained EPSP has a
longer time constant than that of the falling phase of
each EPSP ripple. In this context the vibratory EPSP
ripples and the maintained depolarization can be regarded as "vibratory EPSPs" and "steady EPSP" respectively.
Such a dual classification of fast and slow changes of
the membrane potential could be also explained in the

following way: vibratory EPSPs are elicited by the monosynaptic synchronous transmission of Ia impulses at the
involved α-motoneurone and the steady EPSP by some polysynaptic facilitatory impulses which are so "asynchronous" that no definite "ripples" can be found by the
present mode of recording.

Detailed observation of the vibratory EPSPs reveals
that undulation of EPSP size is always present during
vibration. When the vibratory intensity is superior to
a certain level, the first vibratory EPSP is very large
and the second one small. This tendency is well illustrated in Fig. 3E and F, especially in the latter one.
This abrupt diminution of EPSP could be explained by a
recurrent inhibition, occurring in some other homonymous
motoneurone while the transmission at the penetrated
motoneurone is laterally inhibited (Eccles, Fatt and Koketsu, 1954; Wilson, 1966).

4. Motoneuronal Firing during Vibration

Spikes in the motoneurone occur when the vibratory
intensity is increased beyond a certain level and the
resulting vibratory EPSPs depolarize the motoneurone up
to its firing level as shown in Fig. 4.

It is seen in the figure that successive vibratory
EPSPs intermittently trigger spike generation when a
critical depolarization is attained by temporal summation

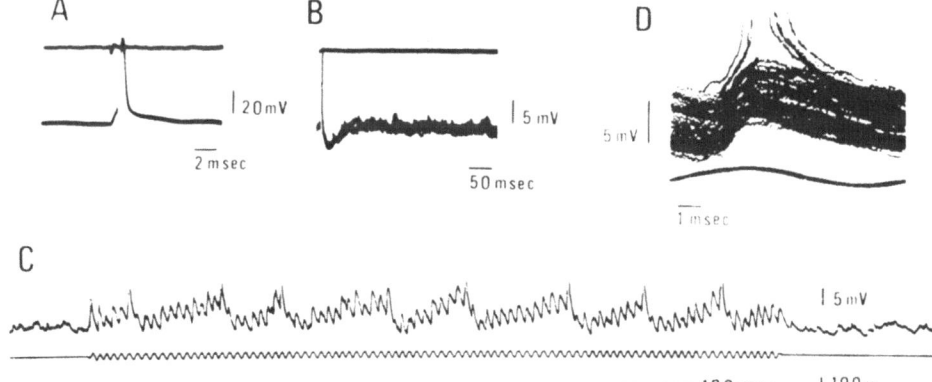

Fig. 4   Cat gastrocnemius motoneurone. A and B show
          orthodromic and antidromic responses respectively.
          Each upper trace shows the dorsal root potential.
          C shows EPSP ripples and motoneuronal spikes
          during 100 Hz vibration. D is superimposed re-
          cords of C at much faster sweeps.

of vibratory EPSPs. It is also an invariable observation that every spike generation occurs at the very
peak of one of the most depolarized vibratory EPSPs. It
becomes therefore natural that the motoneuronal spikes
are separated by the integer multiples of the vibratory
EPSPs, i.e. vibratory cyclic time (Homma et al., 1970).
It can now be argued that the notion of integer multiple
principle repeatedly mentioned in our preceding TVR experiments is verified here by the intracellular time
course of potential change.

The value of the successive integers of interpolat-
ed vibratory EPSP in the sample record, Fig. 4C, is 5,
12, 8, 14, 10, 13, 10 and 10. Since the number of vibratory EPSPs per second precisely coincides with that of
vibratory frequency, 100 Hz, the intervals between motoneuronal spikes can be very easily expressed in milli-
seconds when the number of vibratory EPSPs is multiplied
by ten. A simple, non-sequential inter-spike interval
histogram will give six peaks, the one at 50 msec being
the highest in this sample.

Detailed measurement of Fig. 4C shows a gradual increase of the depolarization needed for motoneuronal
firing. This suggests that an accommodation process is
taking place at the motoneuronal membrane (Araki and
Otani, 1959; Homma, 1966).

One can also notice in Fig. 4C a very gradual upward shift of the intracellular potential. This is probable, though partly due to the effect of temporal summation of the vibratory EPSPs, by means of which such a
slow undulation of the intracellular potential might be
caused by some polysynaptic pathway. This averaged
"steady EPSP" is generated during vibratory stimulation.
Fig. 4D shows the steady EPSP in more details by super-
imposition of much faster sweeps.

5. Decoding Ratio Modifications by Stretching

of the Synergist Muscle

It has already been noticed that the decoding ratio
changes gradually when TVR is tested during concurrent
muscle stretch (Homma et al., 1972). A recording of
intracellular motoneuronal activity is shown in Fig. 5A
where the gastrocnemius motoneurone was penetrated. Spike
initiation is observed only once at the very beginning
of the vibratory stimulation, even though it is followed
by a small steady EPSP. Repetitive spike initiation is,

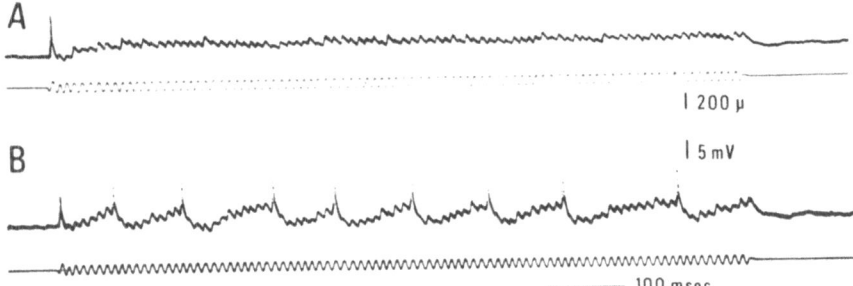

Fig. 5   Gastrocnemius motoneurone. A shows intracellul-
          ar motoneuronal activity during 100 Hz vibra-
          tion, one spike, vibratory EPSPs and steady
          EPSP. B shows repetitive spikes when the soleus
          muscle is stretched.

however, observed when the soleus muscle, the synergist,
is concurrently stretched as shown in Fig. 5B. A slight
change of the resting membrane potential, about 2.5mV
depolarization, is shown as an upward shift of the base
line. Therefore, there is little doubt that the initiation of repetitive excitation in B was achieved by this
upward shift.

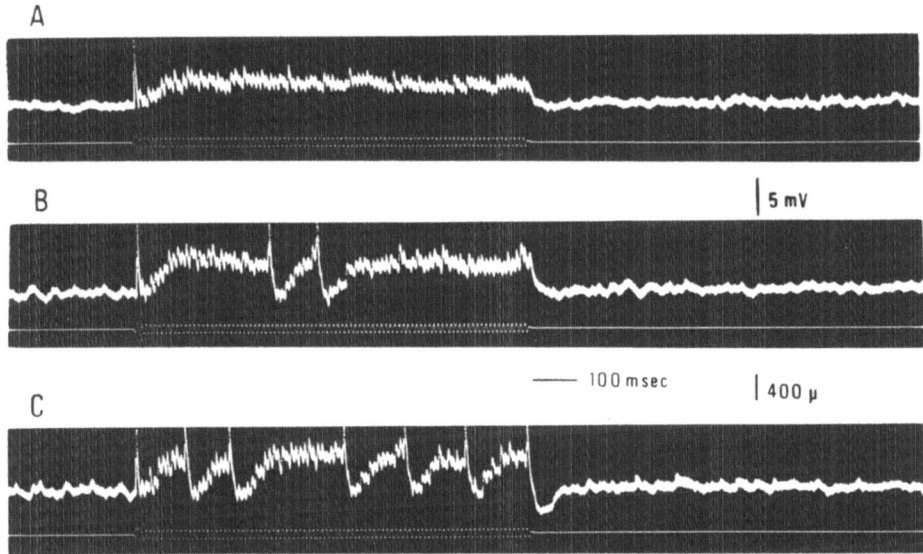

Fig. 6   Gastrocnemius motoneurone. A is the intracellular
          potential change during 100 Hz vibration. B and
          C show the same records when the soleus is
          stretched.

A principle of integer multiples of the cyclic time
of vibration could be applied in the same way to the
spike intervals as clearly seen in B. It could be generally mentioned that the stretch of synergists greatly
increases the decoding ratio (diminution of spike intervals).

It must be noticed again that no appreciable difference in the size of vibratory EPSPs can be found by
between Fig. 5A and B but there is a sizable difference
in the steady EPSP. This means that there is a considerable overlap of some polysynaptic pathway within spinal
cord and that this polysynaptic circuit was also actuated by the synergist stretch and its Ia afferents.

Another sample record from the same experiment is
shown in Fig. 6.

Record A shows the intracellular potential change
when the gastrocnemius muscle only is stretched sinusoidally at 100 Hz. Both vibratory EPSPs and the contingent steady EPSP are generated. Record B shows the same
when the soleus muscle, the synergist, is stretched. A
slight depolarization preliminary to vibratory stimulation can be seen in the upward shift of the base line
with added activation noise (Kolmodin and Skoglund,
1958; Kuno, 1964a,b; Granit, Kellerth and Williams,1964).
A remarkable development of steady EPSP is provoked by
the manoeuvre while the size of the vibratory EPSPs do
not show much difference as compared to the ones of
record A. The development of steady EPSP allows the
motoneurone to fire twice after the initial spike in
record B. A larger stretch applied to the soleus elicits
larger upward shift, activation noise and steep steady
EPSP and a greater number of motoneuronal firing as
seen in the record C. The amplitude of the vibratory
EPSPs again does not show any appreciable change as compared with that in records A and B. As may be judged by
the increased activation noise seen in the base line of
records B and C, a greater amount of high frequency
repetitive discharge must be arriving during synergist
stretch through multineuronal circuit. This added excitation through the interneuronal network should play
an essential role in eliciting the steady EPSP and
resultant spike initiation, since the vibratory EPSPs
do not undergo any remarkable change after stretching
of the synergist.

6. Tonic Vibration Reflex

The intrinsic nature of TVR is expressed in the common characteristic that it appears always as an incremental pattern, especially in the human experiment (Hagbarth and Eklund, 1966a,b). It has been argued (Homma et al., 1971 a,b), that the integer ratio of decoding in the spinal input and output relationship gradually decreases during vibration (Homma et al., 1971 a,b). The above relationship can be simply expressed as follows:

$$MN_f = \frac{1}{n} I_{af}$$

where I_{af}, MN_f and n are: impulse number of Ia afferents and motoneurone per second, and the decoding ratio. The increment of tension during TVR is explained by the gradual but saltatory diminution of n by integers only and the resultant increase of the decoding ratio, 1/n.

Fig. 7 shows another sample of intracellular activity recorded at the gastrocnemius motoneurone during vibratory stimulation of 100 Hz. The motoneuronal spike is followed by a typical after-hyperpolarization which is immediately followed by successive vibratory EPSPs and the steady EPSP.

A

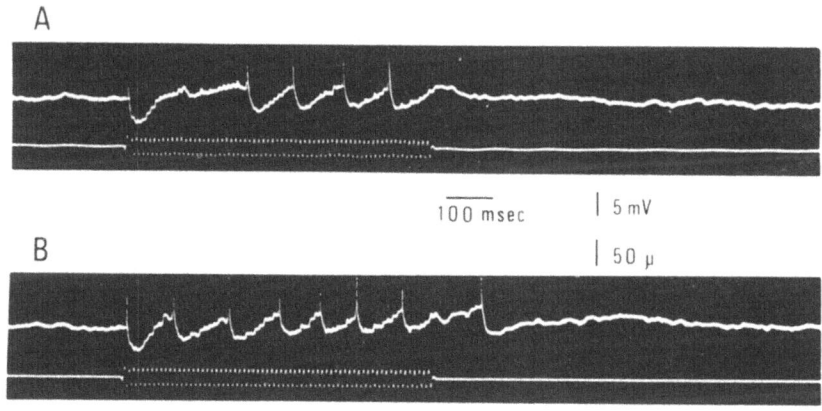

100 msec | 5 mV

B | 50 μ

Fig. 7   Gastrocnemius motoneurone. Intermittent firing is seen during vibratory stimulation at 100 Hz. The motoneurone is firing more frequently at the later phase of the vibratory stimulation. A counteracting influence upon steady EPSP is seen between the first and the second spikes of A.

Intermittent firing occurred whenever the critical
threshold for firing was attained. As seen in the figure
the incremental steady EPSP forced the motoneurone to
fire more frequently at the later phase of the vibratory
stimulation. A more typical time course of such gradually increased firing of the motoneurone is shown in Fig.
7B. Since a gradual increase of motoneuronal firing.i.e.
gradual diminution of the firing interval was observed
only in the presence of the incremental steady EPSP and
of the apparently unchanged size of the vibratory EPSPs,
the tonically increasing tension of TVR may be explained
by the incremental steady EPSP which is supposed to be
effected by an elevated activity of the relevant polysynaptic pathway, due to an integrated post-tetanic
potentiation at the terminal of the interneurones during
vibratory stimulation. An interesting observation which
is noticed in the record of Fig. 7B is that a sustained
depolarization not only continues even after the cessation of vibratory stimulation but also triggers a full
spike. This will be discussed below in detail.

In spite of a developed steady EPSP where impulse
initiation could be expected, a counteracting influence
upon steady EPSP could be observed. For example, an ex-
ceptionally long interval was observed between the first
and the second spikes of Fig. 7A. This suggests a possibility of recurrent inhibition elicited by an adjacent
homonymous motoneurone as already mentioned above. This
counteracting influence is intermittently observed in
the sample record shown in Fig. 8.

The occurrence of counteraction is pointed by the
downward arrows where possible firings of motoneurone
are suspected to be abolished. It is interesting that
such hyperpolarizing deflection occurred almost with
the same temporal undulation as that of depolarizing deflection or spikes. It is very probable that such

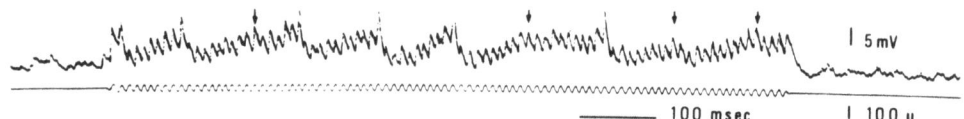

100 msec | 100 µ

Fig. 8   Gastrocnemius motoneurone. Counteracting influ-
         ences upon steady EPSP, expressed by hyper-
         polarizing deflection are pointed by the down-
         ward arrows. Their undulation is temporarily
         the same as that of the spikes.

counteraction is therefore an effect due to some lateral
inhibition actuated by a recurrent neurone, the activity
of which being triggered by the intermittent excitation
of an adjacent homonymous motoneurone because, during
TVR, asynchronous firing of approximately the same repetition rate may be occurring within the involved motor
neurone pool.

    Further detail of the intracellular potential
change during the incremental time course of TVR is
shown in Fig. 9 where 100 Hz vibratory stimuli of 0.9
second duration were repeated 25 times with an interval
of 2 seconds between each.

    Four samples, 6th, 12th, 17th and 21st records,
were selected as indicated by the number in the figure.
Gradual diminution of the membrane potential can be
seen in the figure as judged by the base line. It can be

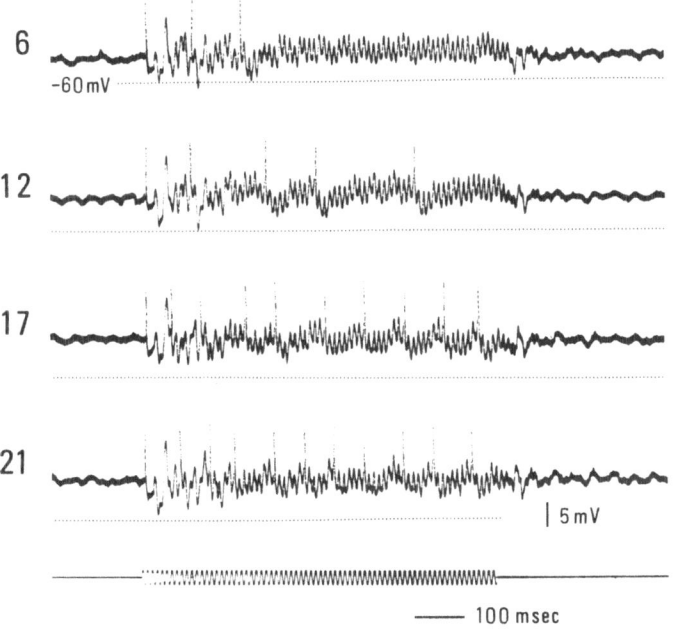

Fig. 9   Gastrocnemius motoneurone. 100 Hz vibratory
         stimuli of 0.9 second duration were repeated
         25 times. Four samples, the 6th, 12th, 17th and
         21st are shown. During the successive vibra-
         tions, both steady EPSP and motoneuronal firing
         increases but the amplitude of the vibratory
         EPSPs is not modified.

also noticed that the steady EPSP is increased too with
repetition of vibratory stimulation while no noticeable
changes occur in the size of the vibratory EPSPs. In
these sample records motoneuronal firing markedly increased from 3 (top record) to 11 impulses (bottom
record). The direct effect for the elicitation of TVR
is attributed to the steady EPSP as suggested by this
experiment.

DISCUSSION

Vibratory stimulation was applied to the skin area
just above the muscle tendon both in the human and
monkey experiments. In the cat experiment muscles were
carefully separated from the neighbouring tissues, the
tendon was also cut at the end and the muscles were
stimulated by longitudinal sinusoidal stretch. In all
experiments vibration was effective for to eliciting a
TVR which could be maintained during the whole period
of vibratory stimulation. A typical time course of TVR
contraction, namely a gradual recruitment of tension was
best observed in the awake human. The time course of
TVR in the slightly anaesthetized monkey was quite different. This difference in the pattern of TVR production
might be due to differences in either the level of con-
ciousness or to the intrinsic difference of the involved
reflex pathways in the monkey. The TVR in the cat could
be well observed in both decerebrate preparation and in
the intact cat under chloralose-urethane anaesthesia.
The TVR is regarded as akin, in nature, to the stretch
reflex. In both cases the primary endings are stimulated
and the Ia muscle afferents excite motoneurones reflex-
ively (Hagbarth and Eklund, 1966a,b). A neural mechanism
responsible for the gradual recruitment of the contraction observed during TVR has been recently suggested,
consisting in a polysynaptic reflex actuated by sustained Ia muscular afferentation during vibration (Fig.
10). This means that the spinal interneurone responsible
for the TVR may be under the influence of post-tetanic
potentiation in order to elicit the TVR effectively
(Kanda, 1972). From the intracellular activity of the
penetrated motoneurone shown above it will safe to
propose that in eliciting the TVR, participation of both
monosynaptic Ia activity and a polysynaptic interneuronal
activity is very probable (Kolmodin, 1957; Eccles,Eccles
and Lundberg, 1960; Tsukahara and Ohye, 1964; Lance,
De Gail and Neilson, 1966). The participation of polysynaptic pathway in a tonic stretch reflex has already

been suggested (Granit, Phillips, Skoglund and Steg, 1957). As already mentioned, the maintained and slowly incremental depolarization is again proposed to be effected through a polysynaptic reflex arc within some segments of the spinal cord and this activity added to the monosynaptic driving should play a very important role.

As present in the section of experimental results the terms of vibratory EPSPs and steady EPSP have been proposed (see Fig.10). The same finding as that of vibratory EPSPs has been already reported in one of our previous reports (Homma et al.,1970). In the present report a relatively high frequency of vibration, 100 Hz, was shown invariably to elicit vibratory EPSPs at a one to one correspondence. The intracellular record of the present experiment further shows a slower potential change, superimposed upon the regular vibratory EPSPs as already expected and shown in a schematic diagram of a preceding paper (Homma et al., 1972). When the critical firing threshold is attained by the summated effect of both vibratory EPSPs and a slower depolarization, partly that of steady EPSP, the firing takes place, without exception, at the very peak of a vibratory EPSP and, therefore, the intervals between spikes are consistent with the integer multiplication principle (Homma et al., 1971a). It is sometimes observed that the superimposed incremental vibratory EPSPs fails to trigger motoneuronal firing although the depolarization level is sufficient for that effect, as indicated by downward arrows in Fig. 8 and Fig. 10. Here, on the opposite, the temporary peak of the undulating depolarization is followed by a relatively low-voltage vibratory EPSPs while the steady EPSP is counteracted by a suspected temporary hyperpolarization. Detailed measurement of the undulation observed ih these vibratory EPSPs in the silent motoneurone (MN1 or 2 in Fig. 10) revealed that there is a very similar time course between the vertical undulation and the spike interval of the firing motoneurone (MN2 or 1). A very similar inhibitory mechanism, therefore, might exist both in the silent and firing motoneurones, provoking a similar time course of motoneuronal behaviour. It is suggested that the intermittent abolition of motoneuronal firing is probably effected by the activity of a Renshaw cell of an adjacent homonymous motoneurone. Such an intermittent abolition of firing can not be explained by the tonic participation of Ia presynaptic inhibition (Eccles, 1964; Gillies, Lance, Neilson and Tassinari, 1969).

When the penetrated motoneurone with the firing
rate of an instantaneous decoding ratio of 1/n receive
lateral recurrent inhibition and the next firing is presumed abolished, the ratio may be reduced to 1/2n(Fig.10).
In the interval when two spikes are presumed abolished,
the decoding ratio will be reduced to 1/3n. It is possible to consider that each homonymous neurone contri-
butes to the lateral recurrent inhibition in the homonymous motor neurone pool. Decoding ratios of 1/2n and
1/3n thus should be regarded to be applicable to two
adjacent neurones alternatively if a very simple model
is considered within a limited space of a pool. Furthermore, it also may follow that the homonymous motoneurones firing at high rates effectively suppress the
motoneurones discharging at low rates (Granit and Renkin, 1961; Kameda, Nagel and Brooks, 1969).

The above assumptions could be a possible explanation of the rhythmic spikes observed during vibratory
stimulation since no other direct observation is available besides that concerning the vibratory EPSPs and
the steady EPSP as investigated in the present experiment. At this moment it is possible to state that the
classical tonic stretch reflex is a temporal and spatial summation of both vibratory EPSPs through monosynaptic transmission and of steady EPSP through polysynaptic
excitation, the latter circuits being mainly responsible
for the incremental activity of TVR by their post-tetanic

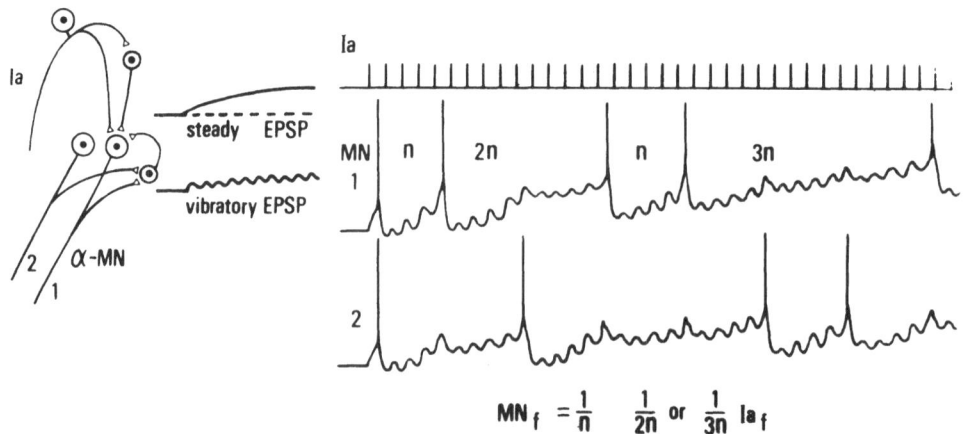

Fig. 10   Schematic diagram showing the sequence of
          events when motoneuronal spikes are triggered
          by the regular incoming Ia discharges during
          vibratory stimulation.

potentiation (Granit et al., 1957) due to vibratory afferents.

The postvibratory steady EPSP which was observed
in the record of Fig. 7B is considered to support the
data of post-vibratory facilitation obtained in the
human experiment. The post-vibratory development of a
steady EPSP can be explained by an enhanced arrival of
facilitatory influence conveyed by some multisynaptic
circuits or a direct arrival of Ia discharge elicited
by mechanical effects of long lasting vibration to the
intrafusal muscle fibers.

The authors express their gratitude to Professor
Shiroh Watanabe for linguistic corrections of the manu-
script. This study was supported in part by a research
grant from the Ministry of Education of Japan.

SUMMARY

Intracellular motoneuronal activity was recorded
in the spinal cord of decerebrate cat. The muscle which
belonged to the motoneurone was sinusoidally stretched
by a vibratory stimulation of 100 Hz.

1. Intracellular recording revealed a 'frequency'
of excitatory postsynaptic potentials (EPSP) precisely
corresponding to that of vibration. The EPSPs are presumably elicited by Ia discharges monosynaptically
transmitted to the penetrated motoneurone and the term
vibratory EPSPs, is suggested.

2. Besides vibratory EPSPs sustained vibratory
stimuli generate a gradual slow incremental depolarization without any change in the size of vibratory EPSPs.
This slow depolarization is supposed to represent a
steady EPSP. The steady EPSP is presumably generated by
some segmental polysynaptic pathway activated during
sustained vibratory stimulation.

3. Motoneuronal firing is triggered whenever a
critical threshold is attained by the vibratory EPSPs
superimposed on the steady EPSP. Therefore the intervals
between motoneuronal spikes are some integer multiples
of the cyclic time of the vibration applied to the
muscle. The firing frequency of a motoneuron is $\frac{1}{n} V_f$

where V_f = vibratory frequency, n = integers, 1, 2, 3,..
n, 1/n = decoding ratio.

4. The hyperpolarization after an initial motoneuronal spike is immediately followed by an increment-
ally depolarizing steady EPSP which lasted throughout
the whole period of vibratory stimulation. Intermittent
counteraction against this steady EPSP was also observed. The counteraction occurring during the incremental
time course of the steady EPSP was supposed to be due
to a lateral inhibition induced by an adjacent homonymous motoneurone. Whenever the firing threshold was
not attained because of the counteraction the decoding
ratio (1/n) decreased as 1/2n, 1/3n and so on.

5. The incremental stretch observed in TVR is presumably due to an increase of the decoding ratio (1/n),
i.e. by a diminution of n.

REFFERENCES

ARAKI, T. and OTANI, T. (1959). Accomodation and local
   response in motoneurone of toad's spinal cord. Jap.
   J. Physiol. 9: 69-83.
BESSOU, P. and LAPORTE, Y. (1962). Responses from primary and secondary endings of the same neuromuscular
   spindle of the tenuissimus muscle of the cat. In:
   "Symposium on Muscle Receptors", ed. Barker, D., pp.
   105-119. Hong Kong : Hong Kong University Press.
BIANCONI, R. and VAN DER MEULEN, J.P. (1963). The res-
   ponse to vibration of the end organs of mammalian
   muscle spindles. J. Neurophysiol. 26: 177-190.
BROWN, M.C., ENGBERG, I. and MATTHEWS, P.B.C. (1967).
   The relative sensitivity to vibration of muscle re-
   ceptors of the cat. J. Physiol.(Lond.). 192: 773-800.
CROWE,A. and MATTHEWS, P.B.C. (1964). Further studies
   of static and dynamic fusimotor fibers. J.Physiol.
   (Lond.). 174: 132-151.
ECCLES, J.C. (1964). "The Physiology of the Synapses".
   Heidelberg: Springer Verlag.
ECCLES, J.C., ECCLES, R.M. and LUNDBERG, A. (1960).
   Types of neurone in and around the intermediate muscle
   of the lumbosacral cord. J.Physiol. (Lond.). 154:
   89-114.
ECCLES, J.C., FATT, P. and KOKETSU, K. (1954). Cholinerg-
   ic and inhibitory synapses in a pathway from motor-
   axon collaterals to motoneurones. J.Physiol. (Lond.).
   126: 524-562.
FUKUDA, K. (1972). Muscular afferent discharges during
   vibration. J.Chiba Med.Soc., in press.

GILLIES, J.D,, LANCE, J.W., NEILSON, P.D. and TASSINARI,
    C.A. (1969). Presynaptic inhibition of the monosynapt-
    ic reflex by vibration. J.Physiol. (Lond.). 205:
    329-339.
GRANIT, R. and HENATSCH, H.D. (1956). Gamma control of
    dynamic properties of muscle spindles. J.Neurophysiol.
    19: 356-366.
GRANIT, R., KELLERTH, J.-C. and WILLIAMS, T.D. (1964).
    Intracellular aspects of stimulating motoneurones by
    muscle stretch, J.Physiol.(Lond.). 174: 435-452.
GRANIT, R., PHILLIPS, C.G., SKOGLUND, S. and STEG, G.
    (1957). Differentiation of tonic from phasic alpha
    ventral horn cells by stretch, pinna and crossed ex-
    tensor reflexes. J.Neurophysiol. 20: 470-481.
GRANIT, R, and RENKIN, B. (1961). Net depolarization
    and discharge rate of motoneurones, as measured by
    recurrent inhibition. J. Physiol.(Lond.).158:461-475.
HAGBARTH, K.-E. and EKLUND, G. (1966a). Motor effects
    of vibratory muscle stimuli in man. In: "Muscular
    Afferents and Motor Control. Nobel Symposium I", ed.
    Granit, R., pp. 177-186. Stockholm: Almqvist and Wiksell.
HAGBARTH, K.-E. and EKLUND, G. (1966b). Tonic vibration
    reflex (TVR) in spasticity. Brain Res. 2: 201-203.
GRÜSSER, O.-J. and THIELE, B. (1968). Reaktionen primär-
    er und sekundärer Muskelspindelafferenzen auf sinus-
    förmige mechanische Reizung. I. Variationen der Si-
    nusfrequenz. Pflüg. Arch. ges. Physiol. 300: 161-184.
HOMMA, S. (1966). Firing of the cat motoneurone and
    summation of the excitatory postsynaptic potential.
    In: "Muscular Afferents and Motor Control. Nobel Sym-
    posium I",ed. Granit, R., pp. 235-244. Stockholm:
    Almqvist and Wiksell.
HOMMA, S., ISHIKAWA, K.. Stuart, D. G. (1970). Moto-
    neurone responses of linearly rising muscle stretch.
    Am. J. Phys. Med. 49: 290-306.
HOMMA, S., KANDA, K., WATANABE, S. (1971a). Monosynapt-
    ic coding of group Ia afferent discharges during
    vibratory stimulation of muscles. Jap. J. Physiol.
    21: 405-417.
HOMMA, S., KANDA, K. and WATANABE, S. (1971b). Tonic
    vibration reflex in human and monkey subjects. Jap.
    J. Physiol. 21: 419-430.
HOMMA, S., KANDA, K., WATANABE, S. (1972). Preferred
    spike intervals in the vibration reflex. Jap. J.
    Physiol. 22: 421-432.
KAMEDA, K., NAGEL, R. and BROOKS, V.B. (1969). Some
    quantitative aspects of pyramidal collateral inhibi-
    tion. J. Neurophysiol. 32: 540-553.

KANDA, K. (1972). Contribution of polysynaptic pathways
   to the tonic vibration reflex. Jap. J. Physiol. 22:
   367-377.
KOLMODIN, G. M. (1957). Integrative processes in single
   spinal interneurones with proprioceptive connections.
   Acta physiol. scand. 40: Suppl. 139.
KOLMODIN, G. M. and SKOGLUND, C. R. (1958). Slow membrane potential changes accompanying excitation and
   inhibition in spinal moto- and interneurons in the
   cat during natural activation. Acta physiol. scand.
   44: 11-54.
KUFFLER, S. W., HUNT, C. C. and QUILLIAM, J.P. (1951).
   Function of medullated small-nerve fibers in mammalian
   ventral roots: efferent muscle spindle innervation.
   J. Neurophysiol. 14: 29-54.
KUNO, M. (1964a). Quantal components of excitatory synaptic potentials in spinal motoneurones. J. Physiol.
   (Lond.) 175: 81-99.
KUNO, M. (1964b). Mechanism of facilitation and depression of the excitatory synaptic potential in
   spinal motoneurones. J. Physiol.(Lond.) 175: 100-112.
LANCE, J. W., de GAIL, P. and NEILSON, R. D. (1966).
   Tonic and phasic spinal cord mechanisms in man. J.
   neurol. neurosurg. psychiat. 29: 535-544.
TSUKAHARA, N. and OHYE, C. (1964). Polysynaptic activation of extensor motoneurones from Group Ia fibres in
   the cat spinal cord. Experientia 20: 628-629.
WILSON, V. J. (1966). Regulation and function of Renshaw
   cell discharge. In:"Muscular Afferents and Motor
   Control. Nobel Symposium I", ed. Granit, R., pp. 317-
   329. Stockholm: Almqvist and Wiksell.

MOTONEURONAL REFLEX RESPONSE TO VIBRATION OF THE CONTRACTING MUSCLE

J. Vučo and Radmila Anastasijević

From the Institute for Medical Research

Beograd, Yugoslavia

INTRODUCTION

It was shown by Matthews (1966), Hagbarth and Eklund (1966) that maintained Ia input lead to a maintained motor output. Anastasijević,Anojčić, Todorović and Vučo (1968) showed that vibrating the tendon of gastrocnemius muscle in decerebrated cats, with an amplitude and frequency that causes selective activation of primary endings of the muscle spindle, produced continuous reflex activity of small alpha motoneurones. In subsequent papers (Anastasijević, Cvetkovič and Vučo, 1971 a, b) evidence was presented that fusimotor stimulation, synchronous with short-lasting repetitive vibration, increased the motoneuronal discharge rate to a larger extent than in the case of continuous vibration of comparable duration. In a recent paper (Anastasijević and Vučo, 1972) further evidence of the influence of the gamma loop activity on spinal alpha motoneurones was presented.

The whole question of the effect of fusimotor stimulation and vibration of the muscle on motoneuronal reflex firing was, in this work, explored in more details. Particular attention was paid to the conditions under which the joint effect of both stimuli provided the spinal motoreurones with the ability to overcome both the central effect of unloading the spindle by extrafusal contraction and the inhibitory influences arising from Golgi tendon organs. A precisely patterned recruitment of fresh motoneuronal units during the

joint action of both stimuli and the presence of facilitation of their reflex discharge, even when a considerable number of gamma-motor fibres are not yet excited,
will be demonstrated.

Such a finding seems to be of particular interest
in relation to the servo hypothesis of the muscle control via the stretch reflex.

METHODS

The technique and procedures used in this work
have been described in detail in three previous papers
(Anastasijević et al., 1968, 1971 a, 1972). The experimental material, presented here, derives largely from
the analysis of 49 motoneuronal units of twenty-five
adult cats, analysed from other point of view in the
previous paper (Anastasijević et al.,1972). Other analysis made on units fired during vibration at different
amplitudes and frequencies supported the conclusion
drawn from the systematic investigation of this group
of motor units.

Peak to peak amplitude of vibration of 50μ for
the frequency of 200 Hz was used throughout the experiments. Stimulation of the peripheral stump of either
the cut ventral root L_7 or S_1 was produced by square
pulses of 500μ sec duration and frequency of 200 Hz.

RESULTS

The Recruitment of Motoneuronal Units during Vibration and Concomitant Fusimotor Stimulation

Cessation of motoneuronal unit firing, as well as
recruitment of new units, may occur within the pool of
motoneurones innervating the gastrocnemius medialis
muscle when either the strength of tetanic stimulus (applied simultaneously with the vibration) changed or when
a stimulus of the same strength was applied either in
absence or in presence of muscle vibration. A pair of
motoneuronal units were "set up" by vibration to discharge tonically (Fig. 1). When the strength of stimulation of the peripheral stump of the cut ventral root
was still in the range to excite only alpha fibres (1
and 1.5 times alpha threshold), falling-out of the units
occurred in a size-dependent order, thus producing a

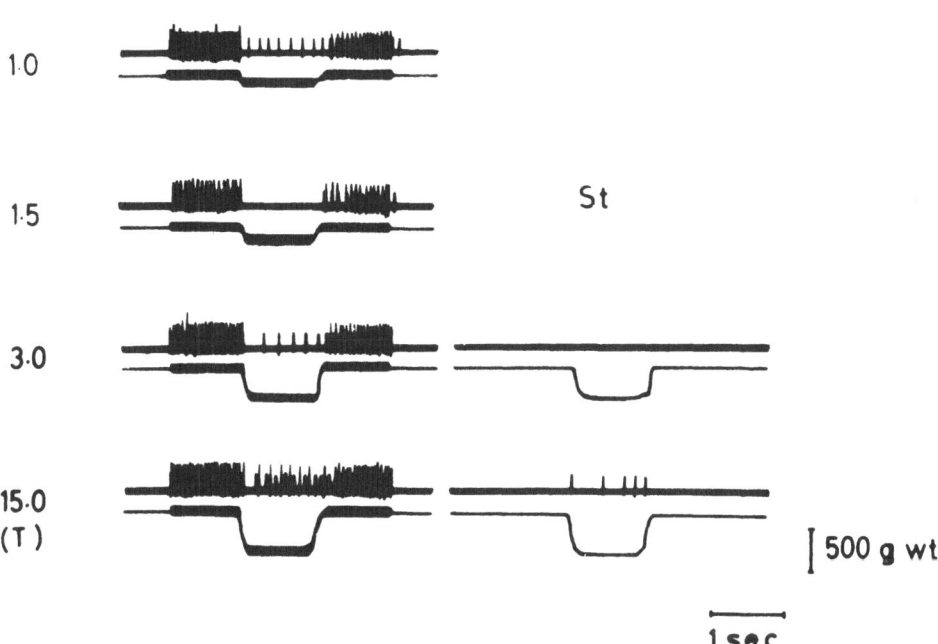

Fig. 1   Reflex response of tonically discharging units
         during vibration and concomitant ventral root
         stimulation (Vi + St, left column). Stimulation
         of the peripheral stump of the cut ventral root
         applied separately (St, right column). Upper
         tracing: motoneuronal reflex spikes. Lower trac-
         ing: isometric myogram; in this figure increase
         of the tension in the muscle appears as a down-
         ward deflection of the oscilloscope beam. In
         this and the following figure thickening of the
         base lines caused by vibration artifact indicat-
         es the duration of vibration. Numbers of the
         left indicate the strength of electrical stimuli
         in terms of multiples of alpha threshold.

pause in the motoneuronal discharge. When a greater number of gamma motor fibres were activated by a further
increase in stimulus strength (3 times alpha threshold),
the pause began to be gradually filled up, first by the
unit with the smaller reflex spike. With a still further
increase in the stimulus strength (15 times alpha thre -

shold), a burst of reflex spikes of the larger unit also
appeared.

   In this experiment 1 sec stimulation was superimposed on the middle period of 3 sec vibration of the
muscle. As the period of stimulation coincided with the
period when vibration already had produced a firing of
the motoneuronal units, one could expect that either
acceleration or diminution of the rate of discharge as
well as recruitment of fresh units during joint application of the stimuli could possibly be related to the
previous reflex activity of the motoneuronal units (Barnes and Pompeiano, 1970; Anastasijević et al., 1971 a,b).
In order to exclude this possibility, in four cats,either
vibration was superimposed on the middle of stimulation
or both stimuli were applied simultaneously. In both
cases the threshold values for reflex firing of motoneuronal units were found to be the same. As it was
desirable to record even the smallest changes in the
rate of motoneuronal reflex firing and moment to moment
recruitment or falling-out of units when the strength of
ventral root stimulation was changed and also to compare then with the values immediately preceding and
following, in further experiments the stimulation was
superimposed on the middle period of muscle vibration
and only rarely both stimuli were applied simultaneously.

        Facilitation of the Reflex Effect of the Joint
Action of Vibration and Fusimotor Stimulation

   Progressive summation of the facilitatory effect
of the joint action of muscle vibration and fusimotor
stimulation occurred when the stimuli were applied simultaneously in a repetitive manner (Fig. 2). Although
the ventral root stimulation (St) alone did not yet produce loop activation of the unit, two reflex spikes appeared during muscle contraction when both stimuli were
applied together (Vi + St, first trial) and their number
increased progressively in each subsequent trial without
any visible reduction of the amount of isometric muscle
tension.

   An example of the reflex effect of a repetitive
series of the stimuli, simultaneously applied, when the
strength of the ventral root stimulation is changed in
a step-like manner, is shown in Fig. 3. At threshold
value for alpha fibres the first trial /I/ in the sequence of stimuli failed to produce the reflex discharge
of the motoneuronal unit. With successive stimuli

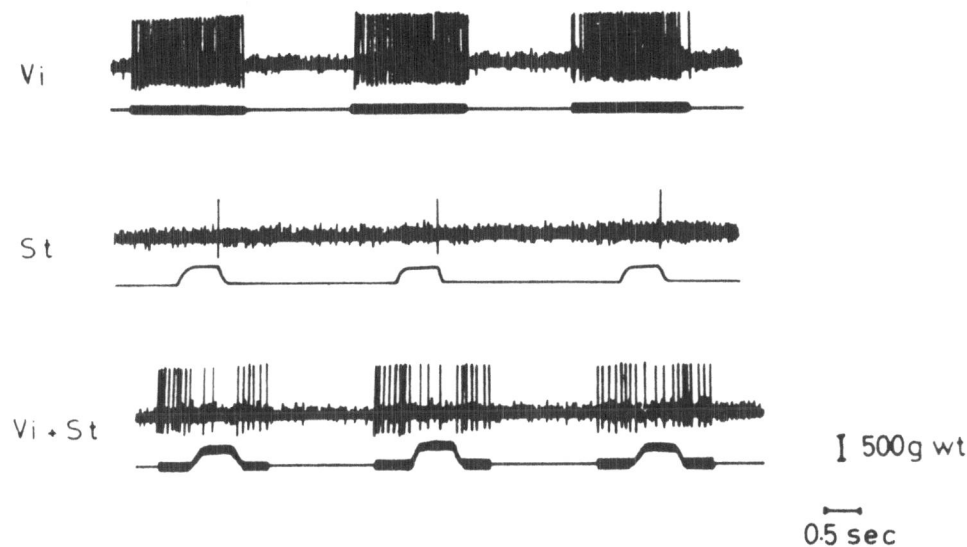

Vi

St

Vi + St

I 500g wt

0.5 sec

<u>Fig. 2</u>   Reflex response pattern of motoneuronal unit
during repetitive vibration (Vi), ventral root
stimulation - 1.7 times alpha threshold (St) and
both stimuli applied together (Vi + St). Upper
tracing: motoneuronal reflex spikes. Lower tracing: isometric myogram. Note that single spikes
visible in the middle row coincide with a sudden
release of muscle tension.

(II-X trials) progressive increase in the reflex response
took part. When the stimulus strength was greater
(1.3 - 2.0 times alpha threshold) the reflex discharge
of the motoneuronal unit occurred already at the first
trials, but each successive trial in the sequences still
produced an increase in number of reflex spikes. With
further increase in the stimulus strength (2.3 times
alpha threshold), the motoneuronal unit fired from the
very beginning of the series of trials in such a manner
as it would do in the absence of any muscle contraction
(Anastasijević et al., 1971 a).

     A more detailed picture of filling-up the pause in
motoneuronal reflex discharge during muscle contraction
when vibration and ventral root stimulation were applied
as a repetitive series is shown in Fig. 4. When the

J. VUČO and RADMILA ANASTASIJEVIĆ

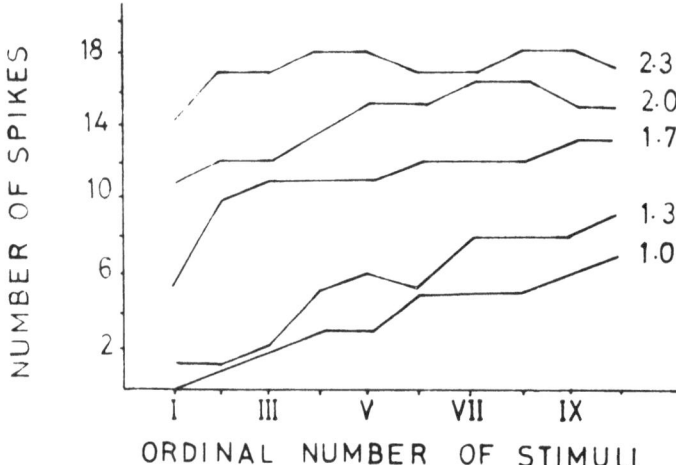

Fig. 3 Number of motoneuronal reflex spikes during
repetitive vibration with fusimotor stimulation
presented as a function of the sequence of
stimulus trials. Ordinate: number of reflex
spikes in a trial. Abscissa: ordinal number of
trials in a series. Duration of trials 1000 msec.
Pauses between trials 1000 msec. Numbers on the
right indicate the strength of electrical
stimuli in multiples of alpha threshold.

strength of ventral root stimulation reached the alpha
threshold, the motoneuronal discharge during the first
trial in the series (I) completely disappeared. With
further increase in the stimulus strength (1.3 - 3.3
times alpha threshold) the reflex firing reappeared, and
its rate gradually increased up to a plateau value. At
the third trials in the series (III), ventral root
stimulation at alpha threshold value caused a decrease
in the number of reflex spikes, but not a complete disappearance of motoneuronal discharge during muscle contraction. With further increase in the stimulus strength,
the increase in motoneuronal firing rate occurred earlier and was always greater than in the first trials of
the series for the same stimulus strength. In each subsequent trial in the sequence (VI, X in this figure),
the fall of the motoneuronal firing rate, caused by muscle
contraction, was less and less marked. Although the progressive decline of the amount of isometric muscle tension took place during repetition of stimulus trials,
this fact cannot be the sole cause of the progressive
increase in motoneuronal reflex discharge: the changes
in muscle tension were noticed only during a few last
trials in the series and only when the stimulus strength
was raised to above 15 times alpha threshold; on the

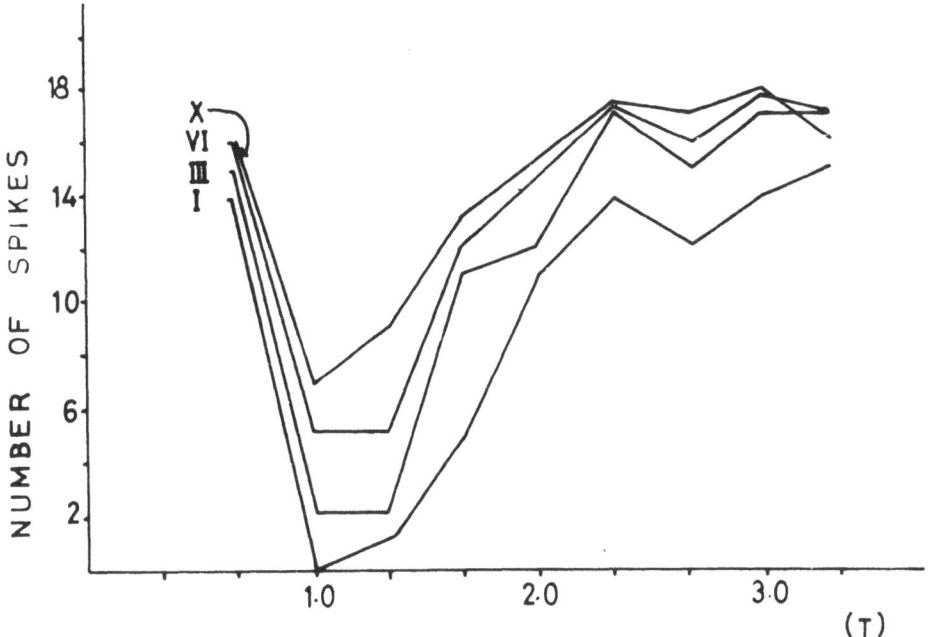

Fig. 4   Number of reflex spikes of the same unit as in
         Fig. 3, but presented as a function of the sti-
         mulus strength. Ordinate: number of reflex
         spikes in a trial. Abscissa: strength of ventral
         root stimulation in multiples of alpha thresh-
         old. Roman figures indicate ordinal number of
         trial in each repetitive series.

contrary, the increase in motoneuronal reflex response
started earlier in the course of repetitive series and
already at stimulus strength at and just above alpha
threshold, and was similar to that found in paralysed
cats (Anastasijević et al., 1971 a).

                         DISCUSSION

     The existence of potential resources of gamma
system influence across the gamma-loop, additional to
those already described (Critchlow and von Euler, 1963;
Granit, Kellerth and Szumski, 1966; Severin, Orlovskij
and Shik, 1967; Anastasijević et al., 1968, 1971 a, b,
1972) has been demonstrated in this work. While the
spindle endings were highly excited by vibration of the
muscle, a step-like rise of the strength of ventral root
stimulation produced a neatly patterned recruitment of
motoneuronal units from the pool. On the other hand a
moment to moment adjustment of the rate of motoneuronal

discharge was seen to occur when both stimuli were applied repetitively, even though fusimotor stimulation
alone did not yet produce "through the loop" activation
of motoneurones. If the gamma loop is fully engaged by
a sufficient stimulus strength and/or its effect is
potentiated by repeating the stimulation, the same pattern and level of motoneuronal reflex response to muscle
vibration may be obtained in presence as in absence of
muscle contraction, the opposing influences of Golgi
tendon organs and of spindles unloading being completely
overwhelmed. These findings represent an additional in
formation concerning the role of gamma system influences
during regulation of muscular movements.

It was not surprising to find again in this work
that the most responsive cells to low-amplitude vibration of the muscle and fusimotor stimulation were the
small, tonically discharging alpha motoneurones. It
would be probably possible, by using a similar experimental technique, to prove that they belong to the so
called S motor units type of gastrocnemius muscle, described by Burke (1967, 1968). One can suppose that,
under the experimental condition described in this work,
a combined activity of both the more powerful and the
low-threshold components of the gamma route for muscle
activation dominated: I. static fusimotor fibres which
increase the vibratory responsiveness of both primary
and secondary endings of muscle spindle (Lennerstrand
and Thoden, 1968; Brown, Engberg and Matthews, 1967);
II. small alpha motoneurones highly responsive to impulses in the large spindle afferents during low-amplitude (50 μ) and high-frequency vibration of the muscle
(Anastasijević et al., 1968).

Nevertheless, the extent of the influence of gamma
loop activity of the reflex response pattern of phasi-
cally discharging or fast motoneurones, when they are
employed for versatility or velocity of movement, could
not be estimated in this work. Another experimental approach to the investigation of the possible regulatory
influence of gamma loop during rapid and strong movements is needed.

SUMMARY

1. Reflex effect of muscle vibration and electrical
stimulation of the distal part of the cut ventral root,
applied simultaneously, was investigated in decerebrated
non-paralysed cats.

2. Disappearance and reappearance of motoneuronal units reflex response to muscle vibration occurred in a size-dependent order when the strength of ventral root stimulation was increased.

3. Increase in motoneuronal firing rate, as well as recruitment of new units during vibration of contracting muscle was caused at stimulus strength still insufficient to fire the units "through the gamma loop".

4. The facilitatory effect of a joint action of muscle vibration and fusimotor stimulation, applied in a repetitive manner, increased progressively in each subsequent trial of a sequence.

5. These results are duscussed from the póint of view of servo-control of muscular contraction.

REFERENCES

ANASTASIJEVIĆ R., ANOJČIĆ M., TODOROVIĆ B. and VOČO J. (1968). The differential reflex excitability of alpha motoneurons of decerebrate cats caused by vibration applied to the tendon of the gastrocnemius medialis muscle. Brain Res., 11:336-346.

ANASTASIJEVIĆ R., CVETKOVIĆ M. and VUČO J. (1971 a). The effect of short-lasting repetitive vibration of the triceps muscle and concomitant fusimotor stimulation on the reflex response of spinal alpha motoneurones in decerebrated cats. Pflügers Arch., 325: 220-234.

ANASTASIJEVIĆ R., CVETKOVIĆ M. and VUČO J. (1971 b). The extensor monosynaptic reflex during repetitive vibration of the muscle. Yugoslav.Physiol.Pharmacol.Acta,, 7: 431-438.

ANASTASIJEVIĆ R. and VUČO J. (1972). Motoneuronal reflex firing during vibration of the muscle and gamma loop activation. Pflügers Arch., 333: 227-239.

BARNES C. D. and POMPEIANO O. (1970). Effects of muscle vibration on the pre and postsynaptic components of the extensor monosynaptic reflex. Brain Res., 18: 384-388.

BROWN M. C., ENGBERG I. and MATTHEWS P. B. C. (1967). The relative sensitivity to vibration of muscle receptors of the cat . J.Physiol.(Lond.), 192: 773-800.

BURKE R. E. (1967). Motor unit types of cat triceps surae muscle. J.Physiol.(Lond.), 193: 141-160

BURKE R. E. (1968). Group Ia synaptic input to fast and slow twitch motor units of cat triceps surae. J.Physiol.(Lond.), 196: 605-630.

GRITCHLOW V. and EULER C. v. (1963). Intercostal muscle
    spindle activity and its γ motor control. J.Physiol.
    (Lond.), 168: 820-847.
GRANIT R., KELLERTH J. O. and SZUMSKI A. J. (1966).
    Intracellular recording from extensor motoneurones
    activated across the gamma loop. J.Neurophysiol.,
    29: 530-544.
HAGBARTH K. E. and EKLUND G. (1966). Motor effects of
    vibratory muscle stimuli in man. In Muscular Afferents
    and Motor Control. Nobel Symposium I, ed. R. Granit,
    pp. 177-186. Almqvist and Wiksell, Stockholm.
LENNERSTRAND G. and THODEN U. (1968). Position and velo-
    city sensitivity of muscle spindles in the cat. III.
    Static fusimotor single-fibre activation of primary
    and secondary endings. Acta physiol.scand., 74: 30-49.
MATTHEWS P. B. C. (1966). The reflex excitation of the
    soleus muscle of the decerebrate cat caused by vibra-
    tion to its tendon. J.Physiol.(Lond.), 184: 450-472.
SEVERIN F. V., ORLOVSKIJ G. N. and SHIK M. L. (1967).
    Work of the muscle receptors during controlled move-
    ment. Biofizika, 12: 502-511.

PHYSIOLOGICAL CHARACTERISTICS OF THE TONIC AND PHASIC MOTOR UNITS IN HUMAN MUSCLES

A. Gydikov and D. Kosarov

From the Institute of Physiology, Bulgarian Academy of Sciences

Sofia, Bulgaria

The alpha-motoneurones constitute an essential element in the system of motor control. The advance of neurophysiology led to the accumulation of abundant information about their properties and functions. There is a certain lack, however, in studies related to the problem of just how the alpha-motoneurones are operating under conditions of natural motor activity, under normal physiological conditions, and particularly in man, where we have an extremely high development of the system of motor control.

One of the possible approaches to this problem is the further improvement of electromyography (EMG) with a view to selective leading off of the impulses from separate motor units (MU). The existing EMG methods provide for observing the activity of separate MU at low and moderate muscle tensions. In an earlier paper /Gydikov and Kosarov, 1972a/ we described a method which provides for selective leading off of impulses from separate MU under high and maximal muscle tension. Since under normal conditions the pattern of discharge of the MU reflects precisely the pattern of discharge of the motoneurones, this method makes it possible to study the functions of different motoneurones in man under natural physiological conditions.

An attempt has been made in the course of the present work to find answers to the following questions:

I. Are there tonic and phasic alpha-motoneurones
in man and what is their respective pattern of discharge.

In experiments on decerebrated cats Granit, Henatsch and Steg (1956a, b) distinguished these two types
of alpha-motoneurones by the method of post-tetanic
potentiation. It has been established that the tonic
alpha-motoneurones have a lower threshold and show a
tendency of continuous low-frequency firing, whereas
the phasic ones have a higher threshold and tend toward
brief high-frequency bursts. That is why it has been
assumed that the tonic alpha-motoneurones are more ap-
proptiate for tonic muscle activity whereas the phasic
ones are more suitable for phasic activity. In the
course of our studies we obtained data in support of
this assumption, which in turn raised new questions:

2. What is the minimum frequency of discharge of
the different alpha-motoneurones innervating different
muscles in man.

The studies carried out by Kernell (1965) have indicated that the minimum frequency of discharge of the
alpha-motoneurones is very closely related to the duration of the afterhyperpolarization. It may be argued
that the afterhyperpolarization determines the duration
of the inter-impulse intervals at minimal frequency of
discharge. On the other hand it has been demonstrated
by Eccles, Eccles and Lundberg (1957a, 1958), Kernell
(1965) and Burke (1967) that the afterhyperpolarization
lasts longer in the tonic alpha-motoneurones than in
the phasic ones.

3. What is the maximum frequency of firing of the
alpha-motoneurones innervating different human muscles,
and to what extent, under normal conditions, the motoneurones operate in the primary and secondary ranges.

Studies carried out by Granit, Kernell and Lamarre
(1966a) have indicated that in the primary range, which
embraces the frequencies of up to about 85% of the
maximum ones, there exists an algebraic summation of the
different alpha-motoneurones inputs. Summing up in the
secondary range takes place at another gain, and frequent deviations from linearity are observed (Granit et
al.1966a).

4. Is there a "rotation" of the alpha-motoneurones
in man and what is the influence of fatigue on the

frequency of discharge of different alpha-motoneurones.
It is generally believed that whole subsets of alpha-
motoneurones are switched alternatively on and off by
a mechanism of control of overall fatigue. It can be
expected that a "rotation" of this type would be observed more clearly at higher muscle efforts, as the
fatigue phenomena would appear more rapidly in this
case.

5. Does recruiment of the alpha-motoneurones depend
on their properties or on the type of input.

In acute experiments on cats it has been found by
Granit, Henatch and Steg (1956a, b) that tonic alpha-
motoneurones are smaller than phasic ones. Henemann
(1957), Henemann, Somjen and Carpenter (1965a, b) established in similar experiments that the recruitment
of the alpha-motoneurones does not depend on the input
but is carried out in accordance with what is known as
the size principle. There is always one and the same
order of recruitment - the larger the alpha-motoneurone
the later its recruitment takes place. It is well known
on the other hand that the tonic alpha-motoneurones are
smaller than the phasic ones. The overall resistance of
the membrane of the small tonic alpha-motoneurones is
higher (Kernell,1965, and Burke,1967), and this factor
is related to the lower threshold. However, it has been
found by Grimby and Hannerz (1968) in man that the sequence of recruitment is subject to change. In repeated
contractions and under the influence of various other
conditions there is a "rotation" of the MUs with the
lowest threshold.

6. Are there inhibitory influences exerted by the
large phasic alpha-motoneurones on the small tonic
alpha-motoneurones.

We know that the recurrent inhibition is more
marked on the tonic alpha-motoneurones (Granit, Pascoe
and Steg, 1957, Granit and Rutledge, 1960). The hypothesis has been advanced by Granit, et al. 1957, Eccles,
Eccles, Iggo and Ito (1961) that the phasic alpha-motoneurones related to rapidly contracting phasic muscle
fibres (Steg,1962, 1964, Burke,1968a, b) exert an in-
hibiting effect on the tonic alpha-motoneurones related
to slowly contracting muscle fibres when rapid movements
are performed.

METHODS

The studies were carried out on healthy Subjects,
male and female, aged between 18 and 44 years with normal EMG's. Twenty persons were initially involved in the
experiments, but in 9 of them we did not succeed to
derivate selectively MU activity. That is why these persons were dismissed and the study was carried out on 11
Subjects. Successful selective recordings were obtained
from a total of 140 MUs whose distribution in different
muscles can be seen in Table I.

A three-channel "Disa" electromyograph was used as
well as the multielectrode shown on Fig.1, consisting
of three small skin bipolar electrodes. For each MU we
took simultaneous recordings of the activity on three
channels, and this made it possible for us to locate
it in the muscle and to determine its size (Gydikov,
Kosarov and Tankov, 1972, Gydikov and Kosarov,1972b).
The location was performed many times during the experiment, and on that basis we were absolutely confident
that it was one and the same MU, provided we obtained
the same co-ordinates and one and the same size.

In some of the studies we recorded the muscle tension by means of a strain-gauge under isometric conditions. The tensiogram was recorded by means of the d.c.
amplifier of the 'Mean Voltage Unit' on one of the
channels. In the course of other experiments we measured
the changes in the joint angle by means of a linear
potentiometer. In this case the displacement output and
the impulse activity were recorded simultaneously.

At low miscle activity the electrodes of the multielectrode of Fig.1 record the impulses of one, two or
several MUs regardless of the place of the multielectrode
along the length of the muscle, provided the lines con-

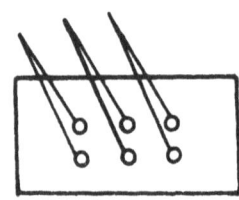

Fig. 1   Multielectrode composed by three bipolar surface
          electrodes with small active surface. Interelec-
          trode distance: 2.5 mm. Distance between the
          pairs of electrodes: 4 mm.

necting the two poles of each electrode pair run parallel to the course of the muscle fibres. In order to obtain a selective recording of impulses from one or
several MUs under high muscle activity, it is necessary
for the multielectrode to be placed in the motor end-
plate area. The precise place depends on the anatomic
characteristics of the muscle investigated and is found
by trial and error. The selective effect is based on the
interrelation of the electrodes and of the active structures. If only one MU is active and recording is done
with a bipolar electrode which is moved through the
motor endplate area along the length of the muscle fibres
(Fig. 2), it will be possible to find such a position
at which the two poles of the electrode will lie at
equipotential points on either side of the motor endplates and the electrode will lead off no potential difference despite the fact that the unit is firing. We
shall refer to this as the zero position of the electrodes. For a large number of MUs the zero position fully
coincides with a transverse line of the muscle surface,
although there are MUs for which the zero position de-
viates more or less from this line. The reason obviously
lies in the position of the motor endplates. Coers and
Woolf (1957) have shown that the motor endplates are
situated approximately along one line, although some of
them may be somewhat aside. When the electrodes are
situated in the common "zero position", at a high muscle
tension it is possible to record activity only from those
MUs whose "zero position" does not coincide with the
common one. Selective recordings are shown on Fig. 3.

        The bulk of the experiments were carried out under
static and uniformly increasing isometric efforts. The
amplified signal from the strain gauge is fed to one of
the beams of a double-beam oscilloscope. The level of the
second one is adjusted so as to provide a reference to
be attained in the static experiments. In the experiments
with continuously increasing isometric tension the

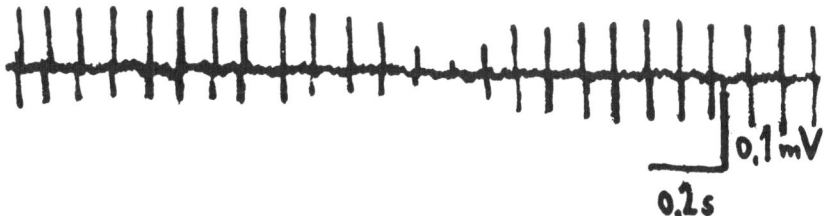

0,1 mV

0,2s

Fig. 2   Passage of a bipolar electrode across the motor
         endplate area of a discharging MU.

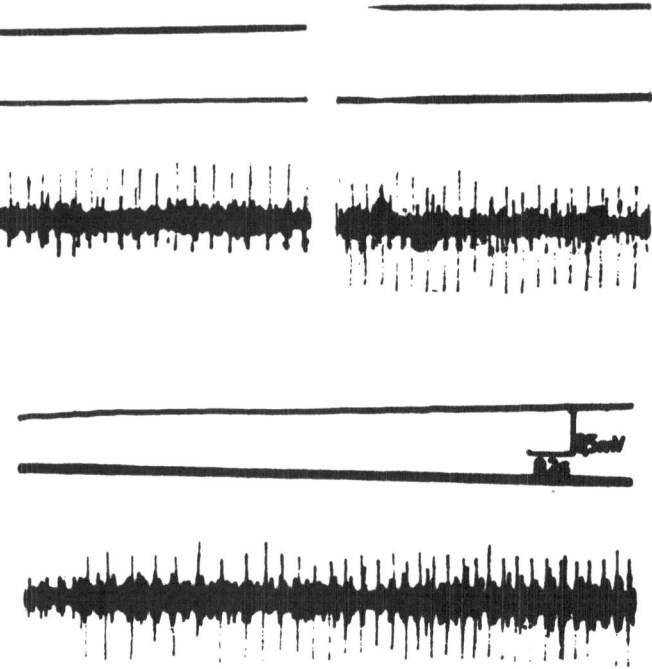

Fig. 3   Selective pick-up of a MU discharge in high
         muscle activity. Above-during maintenance of a
         static effort; below - in a continuous growth of
         the effort.

reference spot is linearly shifted upwards and the Subject is asked to follow it by increasing his muscular
effort. The shift of the spot is performed by means of
a linear potentiometer connected to an electric motor
with controllable speed.

        Whereas most of the experiments involved studies
of the MU discharge under voluntary activation, part of
them dealt with a study of the discharge of various MUs
activated by a stretch reflex. The stretch reflex was
obtained by a sudden increase of a load maintained in
advance, this being done by cutting the string which
holds the counter-load (Fig. 4).

        Special measures were taken to avoid fatigue during
the investigations in which fatigue itself was not an
object of the study undertaken.

        We attempted to study the discharge frequency of an
isolated MU under static load by analyzing 6-sec steady-
state intervals. In other experiments a transient process was provoked by eliciting a stretch reflex or asking

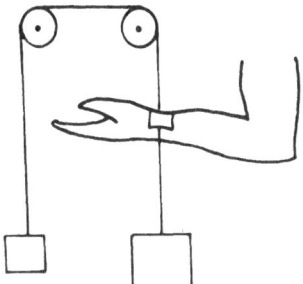

<u>Fig. 4</u>   Experimental set-up in studying a stretch reflex

the Subject to increase stepwise his muscle tension.
The results of 20 such trials were plotted on a fre-
quencygram (Figs.8 and 9).

R E S U L T S

The results of our studies show that the human MUs
can be subdivided in two different types - tonic and
phasic. The first type possesses properties which make
it more suitable for a tonic muscle activity, whereas
the second type is more appropriate for phasic activity.
The different properties of these two types of MUs are
evidenced by a different contribution to the realization
of rapidly growing tensions and a different degree of
fatiguability. These differences are due to a different
relation between the frequency of firing and the level
of static isometric muscle tension. Fig. 5 shows such
relations for several MUs from m.biceps brachii. Two
types can be differentiated very clearly and reliably.
In the first one the frequency rises after recruitment
with the increase in the muscle tension, but reaches a
maximum (this maximum is below 14-15 imp/sec for biceps
brachii), and the further rise in the tension is not
matched by a rise in the frequency. Characteristic of
the second type is a monotonous and almost linear rise
of the frequency until the maximum of the muscle tension.
The figure shows also that the types differ in their
thresholds. Whereas the thresholds of the first type of
MUs are between 0 and 50% of the maximum effort, the
thresholds of the second type of MUs are between 30 and
80% of the maximum effort. It was established by location that the first type of MUs are smaller than the
second one. The equivalent summated potential determined by our method of location (Gydikov et al., 1972, Gydikov and Kosarov, 1972b) for the first type of MUs
varies between 0.1 and 5.0 mV, whereas in the case of
the second type it varies between 2.5 and 11.0 mV.

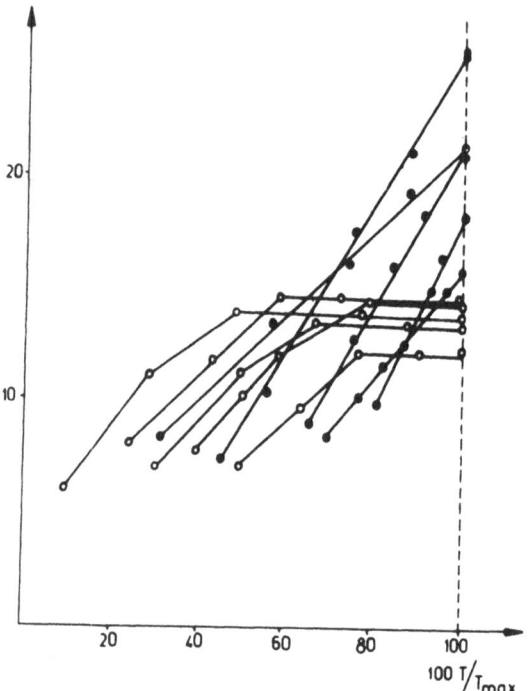

Fig. 5   Relation between the frequency of discharge of
         MUs from m.biceps brachii on the muscle effort.
         Along the abscissa - muscle effort in percentage
         of the maximum effort. Along the ordinate- the
         frequency of discharge of MUs in imp/sec. Empty
         symbols: tonic MUs; full symbols: phasic MUs.

         On the basis of the relation between frequency of
discharge and muscle tension it is possible to calculate
the anticipated change of the frequency of firing for a
given MU when the isometric tension rises at a particular constant rate. Fig. 6 shows the calculated curves
for a MU of the first type and for a MU of the second
type. These curves are compared with experimental data.
We can see that the frequencies are higher than predicted for the second type of MUs during the entire reaction,
whereas for the first type this is the case only in the
beginning. The reason is that the MUs of the first type
reach their maximum frequency of firing very quickly.
Consequently, both types of MUs contribute to the growth
of the muscle tension, but the contribution of the first
type of MUs is insignificant and it occurs only at the
beginning of the dynamic reaction. On that basis it may
be advanced that the second type of MUs is more essential
for the muscle effort in phasic movements.

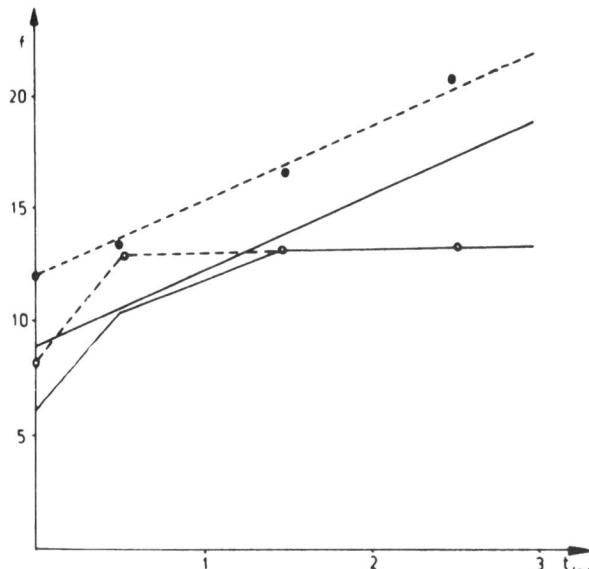

<u>Fig. 6</u>   Comparison between calculated and experimental
          curves for the frequency of discharge of MU
          upon uniform growth of the muscle effort. Dotted
          lines:calculated curves. Solid lines:experiment-
          al curves. Empty symbols; tonic MUs; full sym-
          bols: phasic MUs.

     The first type of MUs shows no essential change in
the frequency of discharge after continuous isometric
contractions. Even 30 minutes of firing cause no change
in the frequency characteristic for a given tension.
The MUs of the second type are easily fatiguable. Fig.7
shows the frequency changes, namely, an initial increase,
a phase of slow-down and the cessation of the discharge.
These changes develop at different rates and they take
several seconds at high frequency. Very probably, at
least part of this difference in the behaviour of the
two types of MUs is due to the difference in the frequency - tension diagram. The low maximum frequency for
the first type of MUs is probably a factor which pro-
tects them against fatigue. Due to the rapid fatiguability of the MUs of the second type they are not suitable for continuous operation.

     The first type of MUs can be called tonic. They
have a lower threshold, they are smaller and relatively
not fatiguable: on that account they are more suitable
for tonic conditions of operation. They contribute little
to the rise of muscle tension during dynamic reactions.
The second type of MUs may be called phasic. They have
a higher threshold, are larger and more readily fatigu-

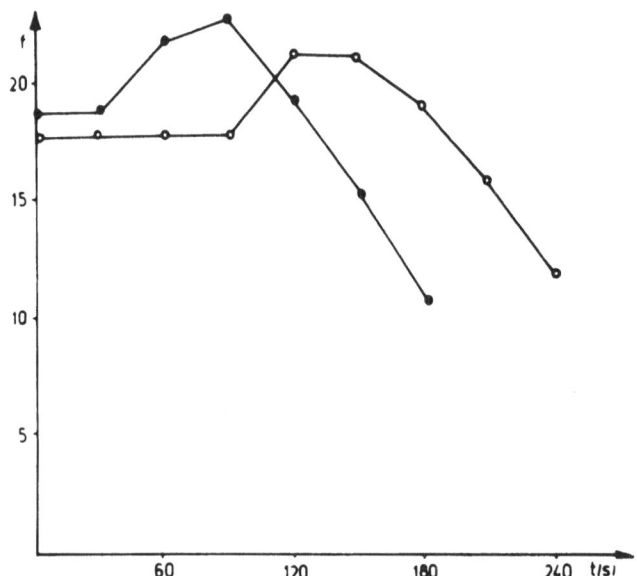

Fig. 7   Frequency of discharge of two phasic MUs during
          high muscle effort maintained on one and the
          same level. Along the abscissa - time in seconds;
          along the ordinate - frequency of discharge
          (imp/sec).

able. Under dynamic conditions they contribute essentially to the increase of the muscle effort. According
to our studies, however, both the tonic and the phasic
MUs participate in tonic isometric contractions and in
phasic isometric contractions.

        Particular attention was paid in the course of our
studies to the minimum frequency with which a given MU
can fire in a stable manner. It turned out that this
frequency is lower for the tonic MUs compared with the
phasic ones, although the difference is not very im-
pressive. The average value for tonic MUs in the human
biceps is 7 imp/sec, while for the phasic MU it is 8.5
imp/sec. This difference is statistically significant
at a level of significance $p < 0.001$. The minimum frequencies of the investigated tonic MUs in m.biceps
brachii vary from 6 to 8 imp/sec, whereas for the phasic MUs the minimum frequency is between 7 and 9.5 imp/
sec.

        One interesting fact is the relatively low maximum
frequencies of the MUs in man under different isometric
tension. They are the highest in the muscles of the
head, lower in the muscles of the arm, and the lowest
in the muscles of the legs (Table I).

T A B L E   I

Number of tonic and phasic motor units investigated and
their maximum frequencies at static isometric tensions
in different human muscles

Muscle	Number of MUs Studied	Number of tonic MUs	Max.freq. of tonic MUs	Number of phasic MUs	Max. freq. of phasic MUs
Orbicularis oculi[*]	12	0	-	12	27-38
Orbicularis oris	11	2	13-16	9	13-33
Masseter	15	4	12-17	11	8-30
Biceps brachii	56	29	11-15	27	11-25
Abductor dig.V	9	3	13-15	6	15-23
Interosseus dors.I (manus)	8	5	12-15	3	12-19
Tibialis anterior	10	3	8-11	7	9-17
Flexor hall.br.	20	10	6-11	10	8-15
Abductor hall.	11	4	7-10	7	7-13

[*]Incomplete   isometric conditions.

        However, when the frequency rises abruptly during
a transient process it is possible to observe higher
frequencies. Fig. 8 shows such transient processes for
one tonic and for one phasic MU during a stretch reflex.
On Fig. 9 the transient processes were observed upon
a stepwise voluntary increase of the isometric tension.
Both figures show the differences in the transient processes of the two types of MUs. Furthermore it can be
observed that during a transient process the frequency
of discharge can be appreciably higher than the maximum
frequency which is observed in the same muscle under
static isometric conditions. On the average for the
investigated MUs in the biceps the maximum frequency in
a steady-state discharge is 73% of the maximum frequency
in a transient process for the tonic ones and 62% for
the phasic ones.

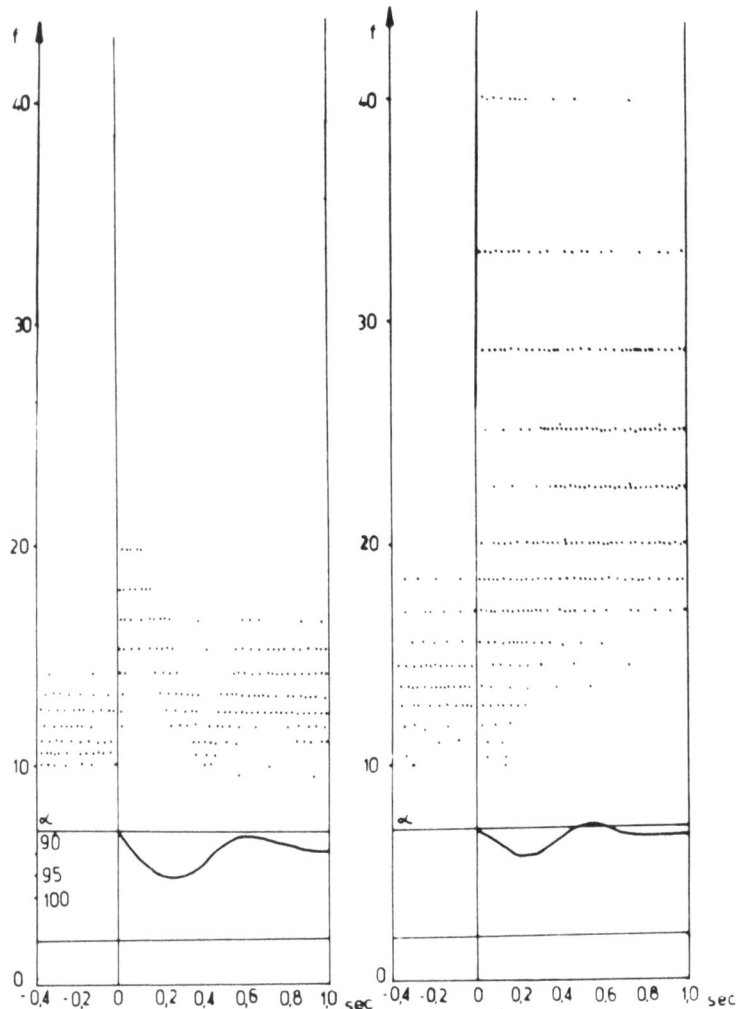

Fig. 8   Transient discharge of MUs from m.biceps brachii
          under stretch reflex. To the left: a tonic MU;
          to the right - a phasic MU. Along the abscissa:
          time in seconds. Along the ordinate: above:
          frequency of discharge in imp/sec, below -
          changes in the joint angle of the elbow in
          stretch reflex eliciting.

     Still higher frequencies are observed when new
tonic MUs are recruited in the stretch reflex or during
a stepwise voluntary rise of the muscle tension. In the
average for the investigated tonic MUs in the biceps
the maximum frequency in a steady-state activation con-
stituted only 58% of the maximum frequency in the transient process from rest toward activity.

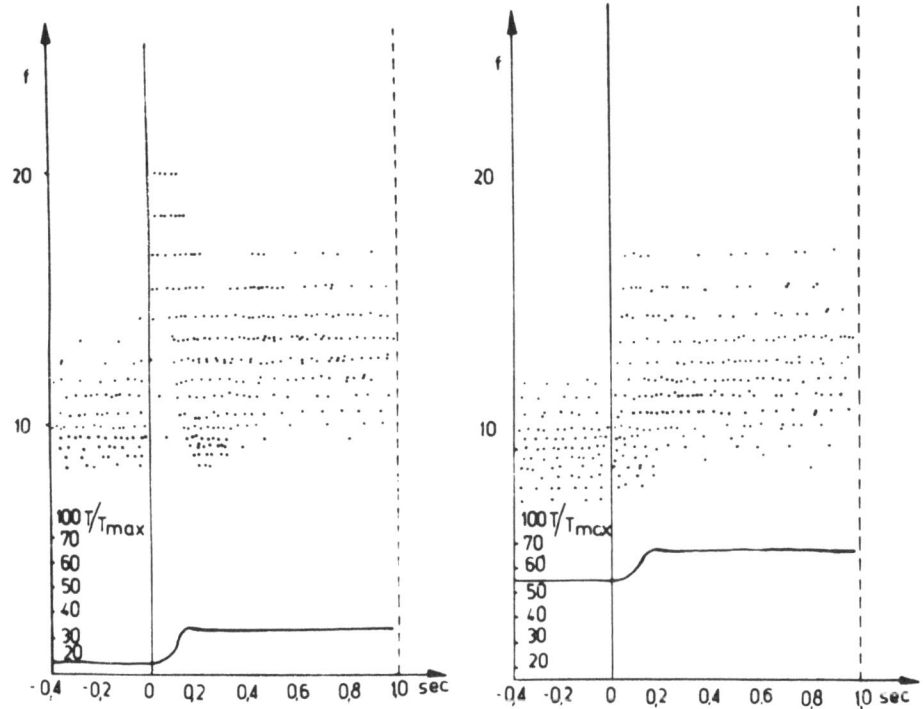

Fig. 9   Transient discharge of MUs from m.biceps
         brachii upon a stepwise voluntary increase of
         the isometric muscle effort. Along the ordinate,
         below: the changes in isometric muscle effort.
         The rest, as in Fig. 8.

        Figures 8 and 9 indicate that the tonic and phasic
MUs behave very differently during a transient activation. In tonic MUs this process evidences an initial
rise in the frequency, a phase of lower frequency, a
secondary rise, and a passage toward a steady-state.Typ-
ical for the transient process of the phasic MUs is a
temporary increase of the standard deviation of the
inter-impulse intervals prior to the transition towards
the new steady-state level, this being particularly
marked during a stretch reflex. We have never observed
in our experiments a drop in the frequency of discharge
or an inhibition of a given MU as a result of the recruitment of other MU during the stretch reflex. The
recruitment of new MU was matched by increased frequency
of discharge of the investigated unit, both in the
transient and in the steady-state process, or only in
the transient process if the unit was a tonic one and
discharge at maximum frequency. This has been established more concretely for the discharge of tonic MUs upon
the recruitment of phasic MUs.

We found no substitution of certain MUs with others ("rotation") during our studies under static isometric conditions. However at a high muscle tension the fatigue does not set on simultaneously in the individual phasic MU (Fig. 7). Obviously, the increase in the frequency of discharge of the MUs is a compensating phenomenon aiming to preserve the necessary tension, despite the fact that other units are operating at lower frequency or have discontinued their discharge.

Upon repeated contraction and relaxation of the muscle the sequence of recruitment may be changed. The experiments in this direction were carried out on m. tibialis anterior and m.biceps brachii.

Particular attention was paid to the rank order of recruitment of the first three MUs. The sequence actually turned out to be variable. It was established upon location that these MUs are very small by their summated equivalent potential.

The size of the motor units evaluated upon location correlates with the average threshold. The threshold in its turn undergoes changes upon repeated contractions. These changes are not in one direction for the individual MU, and as a result of that the sequence of recruitment changes also. However, a change in the sequence of recruitment of two MUs is possible only when their thresholds are close. There is a relation, as shown on Fig. 10, between the difference in the average values of the summated equivalent potential and the probability of the lower threshold MU being activated earlier. The greater the difference in the sizes of two MUs, the greater the probability of the smaller MU being activated first. When the difference exceeds a critical value the smaller MU is always the first to go into action.

D I S C U S S I O N

There can be little doubt that in the human muscle coexist two types of MUs: tonic and phasic MUs. Among the typical features on which is based this distinction, we find: a particular relation between the frequency of firing and the muscle tension (presence or absence of saturation frequency), degree of fatiguability, contribution to the dynamics of tension rise, and transient processes in voluntary activation and in the stretch reflex. Other characteristics do not lead to such a sharp differentiation and are rather continuously distributed. Such are the threshold, the size and

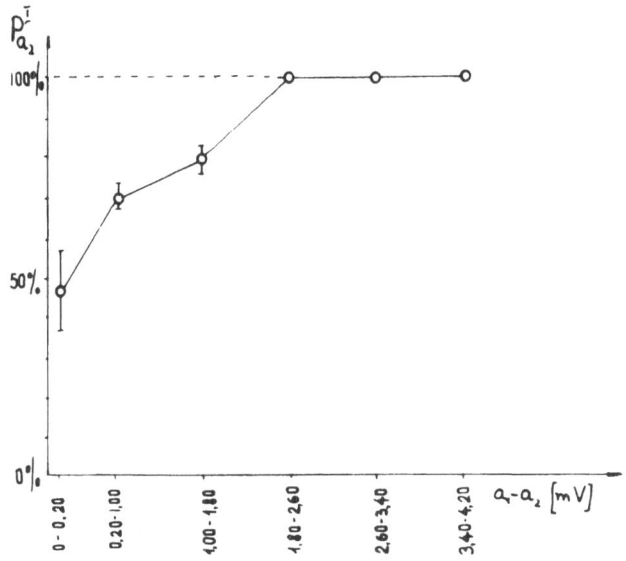

Fig. 10   Relation between the difference of the average
          values of the summated equivalent potential
          for two MUs and the probability of the lower-
          threshold MU entering into action first with
          the increase of the muscle effort. Along the
          abscissa: the difference between the average
          values of the summated equivalent potential of
          the two MUs; along the ordinate: the probability
          of the lower-threshold MU being activated first.

the minimum frequency of firing. Besides that the properties which delineate these two sub-sets are not always convergent. There are some MUs which are tonic according to the frequency - tension criterion, but are
highly fatiguable.

     Confirmation was obtained for the expectation that
the minimum frequency of a stable discharge will be
lower for the tonic MUs, although the difference was
not as great as expected. It may be that under the natural conditions of functioning the duration of the afterhyperpolarization is not the sole factor determining
the minimum frequency. Otherwise it would be necessary
to assume that the difference in this duration for the
tonic and phasic alpha-motoneurones in man is not as
great as it is in cats.

     The fact that the maximum frequency of steady-state
firing constitutes 58 to 73 per cent of the maximum frequency in transient processes is an indication that in
steady-state the alpha-motoneurones in man operate in

the primary range. From the studies carried out until
now it is difficult to assess the degree to which, in
transient processes, the alpha-motoneurones in man operate in the primary range and the degree to which they
operate in the secondary range.

Solving the problem as to the range in which the
alpha-motoneurones are operating under natural conditions is of essential importance for understanding better the processes of control. When both the primary and
the secondary ranges of discharge are being used, the
control signals take account of the changes in the properties of the alpha-motoneurones in transition from
one range into the other. The relatively low maximum
frequencies even in transient processes indicate that
perhaps the entire working range of the frequencies of
the alpha-motoneurones is the primary one. This can be
assumed with a high degree of probability at least for
the steady-state discharges. The saturation frequency of
discharge of the tonic MUs is probably due to a number
of different factors, namely, longer afterhyperpolarization, more marked recurrent inhibition, and inhibition
caused by the Ib afferents. There are experimental data
in support of the view about the role played by recurrent inhibition in stabilizing the frequency of the
motoneurones.

Under normal conditions we did not observe the
assumed by Granit, et al. (1957), Eccles et al. (1961)
recurrent inhibition of the tonic alpha-motoneurones by
the phasic ones during a rapid phasic stretch-reflex.
The small tonic MUs not only participate in the phasic
movements but, as can be seen from Fig. 9, they are the
ones which adjust finely the dynamics of the muscle
force for a more precise performance of the movement.
In the experiments shown on Fig. 9 the Subject investigated tried to provide with maximum speed a strictly
determined rise of the muscle tension. However, the ef-
fector organ exhibits different degrees of inertia, internal friction, and elasticity. Prompt action and precision may be attained provided the control signals are
changed several times. As can be seen from the figure,
such phases of rise and drop in the frequency are observed only in the transient process of the tonic MUs.
The same sequence is elicited by the stretch-reflex as
well (Fig. 8). It was established that the fine control
in both voluntary and reflectory reactions utilizes the
tonic MUs which are probably innervated by tonic alpha-
motoneurones. These data are not in agreement with the

hypothesis advanced by Tokizane and Shimazu (1964) that
the tonic MUs are mainly used for the spinal control of
movements. According to the data obtained by us, the
phasic MUs produce mainly the crude muscle force, while
the precision of the movement, be it voluntary or reflex,
is determined by the tonic MUs. Obviously, in order to
realize these functions of the tonic MUs it is necessary
to assume that they are provided both with more complex
connections at the spinal level and with greater possibilities for cortical control. It is well known, on the
one hand, that the primary afferents of the muscle spindles have a much higher monosynaptic effect on the tonic
alpha-motoneurones (Granit, et al., 1956a, Eccles et al.,
1957, 1958, Granit et al., 1966, Burke, 1968a, b) and that
the recurrent inhibition is more marked in relation to
the tonic alpha-motoneurones (Granit et al., 1957, Granit
and Rutledge, 1960). On the other hand the attempts at
voluntary control of the discharge of individual MU
(Harrison and Mortensen, 1960, Basmajian, 1963) are successful precisely with the small tonic alpha-motoneurones
whose discharge is accessible for investigation by the
conventional EMG methods. Our data show the differences
in the transient processes of the tonic and phasic MUs
at different conditions. The significance of the rate
of muscle contraction for the character of these processes is familiar (Gurfinkel, Mirskyi, Tarko and Sur-
guladze, 1970, Gydikov and Kosarov, 1972a). The new approach applied in the study of the transient processes,
namely, outlining the average changes of the frequency
by superposition of many reactions opens new prospects
for a detailed study of this problem.

The studies undertaken yielded a series of results
relative to what is known as the size principle in the
recruitment of MUs and to the possibility of "rotation". It was found that the size of the MU, which probably corresponds to the size of the respective alpha-
motoneurones, is related to the threshold, i.e. the
tension of the muscle at which a new MU is activated.
However, the thresholds can vary within certain limits.
That is why, the smaller the difference in the average
values of the size of two MUs, the higher the probability of a change taking place in the sequence of their
recruitment in repeated muscle contractions. Consequently, the size is not the sole factor determining the
sequence of the recruitment, although it is an essential one. These results are in agreement with the data
obtained by Person (1972). As regards the sequence of
recruitment of MUs with the lowest threshold, according
to our studies the so-called A, B and C units (after
Grimby and Hannerz, 1968) are always small, tonic MUs.

The opinion expressed by these authors that the A unit
can be a kinetic one is obviously unconvincing. In order
to establish that a MU is a kinetic one it is necessary
to undertake a study of the continuous discharge under
steady-state conditions. According to the data presented
by Grimby and Hannerz themselves (1968) they did not
possess such series of impulses and could not have performed the study they maintain to have carried out.

In addition to changes in the threshold, phenomena
similar to "rotation" are observed in fatigue of the
phasic MUs. When the task is to maintain a particular
muscle tension, the reduction in the frequency of part
of the MUs as a result of fatigue leads to a compensatory
rise in the frequency of another part of the units.
Never, however, provided there are no phenomena caused
by fatigue, have we observed any "rotation", i.e. substitution of the activity of one MU with the activity of
another MU.

C O N C L U S I O N S

1. There are two types of MUs in human muscles -
tonic and phasic ones. The tonic MUs are small, low-
threshold, and they reach a saturation frequency of discharge with the rise of the tension. They do not develop
fatigue, their minimum frequency is lower, and they
contribute little to the dynamic component of the muscle
force though they are of great significance for the line
adjustment of the muscle to its motor task. The phasic
MUs are bigger, with a higher threshold, and they provide an almost linear rise of the frequency with the
increase of the muscle tension. They are readily fatiguable, their minimum frequency of firing is higher and
they contribute to a significant extent to the dynamic
component of the muscle force though they are of no
great significance to the fine adjustment to the motor
task.

2. In a steady-state and under natural conditions
the MUs operate at relatively low frequencies, probably
in the primary range.

3. The size of the MUs which probably coresponds
to the size of the alpha-motoneurones is an important
factor, though not the only one, determining the sequence of recruitment.

R E F E R E N C E S

BASMAJIAN J.N. (1963). Conscious control of single
  nerve cells. New Scientist, 20: 662-664.
BURKE R.E. (1967). Motor unit types of cat triceps surae
  muscle. J.Physiol.(Lond.), 193: 141-160.
BURKE R. (1968a). Group Ia synaptic input to fast and
  slow twitch motor units of cat triceps surae. J.Physi-
  ol.(Lond.), 196: 605-630.
BURKE R.E. (1968b). Firing patterns of gastrochemius
  motor units in the decerebrate cat. J.Physiol.(Lond.).
  196: 631-655.
COERS C. and WOOLF A.L. (1957). The innervation of
  muscle. pp. 6-7, pp 14-20, Oxford, Blackwell.
ECCLES J.C., ECCLES R.M., IGGO A. and ITO M. (1961).
  Distribution of recurrent inhibition among motoneurones.
  J.Physiol.(Lond.), 159: 479-499.
ECCLES J.C., ECCLES R.M. and LUNDBERG A. (1957a). Durations of afterhyperpolarization of motoneurones supplying fast and slow muscles. Nature (Lond.), 179:
  866-868.
ECCLES J.C., ECCLES R.M. and LUNDBERG A. (1957b). The
  convergence of monosynaptic excitatory afferents onto
  many different species of alpha motoneurones. J.Phys-
  iol.(Lond.), 137: 22-50.
ECCLES J.C., ECCLES R.M. and LUNDBERG A. (1958). The
  action potentials of the alpha-motoneurones supplying
  fast and slow muscles. J.Physiol.(Lond.), 142: 275-
  291.
GRANIT R., HENATSCH H.-D., and STEG G. (1956a). Differentiation of tonic from phasic extensor motoneurones by post-tetanic potentiation. J.Physiol.(Lond.),
  133: 12-13.
GRANIT R., HENATSCH H.-D. and STEG G. (1956b). Tonic
  and phasic ventral horn cells differentiated by post-
  tetanic potentiation in cat extensors. Acta physiol.
  scand., 37: 114-126.
GRANIT R., KERNELL D. and LAMARRE Y. (1966). Algebraical
  summation in synaptic activation of motoneurones firing within the "primary range" to injected currents.
  J.Physiol.(Lond.), 187: 379-399.
GRANIT R., PASCOE J.E. and STEG G. (1957). The behaviour
  of tonic α and γ motoneurones during stimulation of
  recurrent collaterals. J.Physiol.(Lond.), 138: 381-
  400.
GRANIT R. and RUTLEDGE L.T. (1960). Surplus excitation
  in reflex action of motoneurones as measured by recurrent inhibition. J.Physiol.(Lond.), 154: 288-307.
GRIMBY L. and HANNERZ J. (1968). Recruitment order of
  motor units on voluntary contraction: changes induced

by proprioceptive aferent activity. J.Neurol.Neurosurg.
  Psychiat., 31: 565-573.
GURFINKEL V.S., MIRSKYI M.L., TARKO A.M. and SURGULAD-
  ZE T.D. (1972). The work of the motor units in man
  upon initiation of the muscle tension. (in Russian).
  Biofizika, 17: 303-310.
GYDIKOV A. and KOSAROV D. (1972a). Studies on the activ-
  ity of the alpha-motoneurones in man by means of new
  EMG methods. In: Neurophysiology in Man. Proceedings
  of the International Symposium on Neurophysiology in
  Man, Paris, July 20-22,1971. Amsterdam, Excerpta
  Medica.
GYDIKOV A. and KOSAROV D. (1972b). Extraterritorial
  potential field of impulses from separate motor units
  in man's muscles. Electromyography, 12: 283-305.
GYDIKOV A., KOSAROV D. and TANKOV N. (1972). Studying
  the alpha-motoneurone activity by investigating motor
  units of various sizes. Electromyography, 12: 99-117.
HARRISON V.F. and MORTENSEN O.A. (1960). Identification
  and voluntary activation of low-threshold motor units.
  Anat.Rec., 136: 207.
HENNEMAN E. (1957). Relation between size of neurones
  and their susceptibility to discharge. Science. 126,
  (3287) : 1345-1346.
HENNEMAN E., SOMJEN G. and CARPENTER D.O. (1965a). Functional significance of cell size in spinal motoneurones.
  J.Neurophysiol., 28: 560-596.
HENNEMAN E., SOMJEN G. and CARPENTER D.O. (1965). Excitability and inhibitability of motoneurones of different sizes. J.Neurophysiol., 28: 597-620.
KERNELL D. (1965). The limits of firing frequency in
  cat lumbosacral motoneurones possessing different
  time course of afterhyperpolarization. Acta physiol.
  scand., 65: 87-100.
PERSON R.S. (1972). Motoneurone's pool and motor control.
  p.4. In: IV International Biophysics Congress. Abstracts of contributed papers, Moscow.
STEG G. (1962). The function of muscle spindles in
  spasticity and rigidity. Acta neurol.scand. 38: 53-59.
STEG G. (1964). Efferent muscle innervation and rigidity. Acta physiol.scand., 61, suppl.225.
TORIZANE T, and SHIMAZU H. (1964). Functional differentiation on human skeletal muscle. (Corticalization and
  spinalization of movement), Springfield,
  Ill. Charles C.Thomas.

PYRAMIDAL AND EXTRA-PYRAMIDAL CONTROL ON MAMMALIAN

ALPHA MOTONEURONES

A. I. Shapovalov

From the Laboratory of Physiology of the Nerve
Cell, Sechenov Institute of Evolutive Physio-
logy and Biochemistry
Leningrad, USSR

Cerebral control of movements in mammals is ac-
complished by the two basic descending systems: the
cortico-spinal or pyramidal and the brain stem-spinal
or extrapyramidal system. The phylogenetically more ancient descending projections originating from brain
stem nuclei developed already in inframammalian vertebrates. However, no definite signs of a pyramidal
system has been reported outside the mammalian world.
The corticospinal tract connects the pyramidal neocort-
ical neurones with the spinal motor centres and extensive work of Kuypers (1960) suggests that direct
monosynaptic connection between pyramidal tract fibers
and alpha-motoneurones may be a special feature of
primates not shared by other mammals. The direct projection of the pyramidal tract to motoneurones becomes
increasingly prominent throughout the primate series to
man and is supposed to be especially advantageous for
the fine control of skilled discrete movements.

For a better understanding of the functional role
of supraspinal motor control and the trends of its
evolution it would be of importance to compare the properties and synaptic organization of the main descending
systems in animals of different degree of encephalization. The present analysis based on local electrical
stimulation of different brain structures and recording
from impaled motoneurones belonging to the hind-limb
summarizes the data obtained in rodents (white rat),
carnivores (cat) and primates (Rhesus monkey).

Brain Stem-Spinal Projections

The synaptic effects elicited in lumbar motoneurones
of different mammals by stimulation of the ponto-medull-
ar reticular formation include poly-, di- and monosynaptic EPSPs, poly- and disynaptic IPSPs. A most striking
analogy exists between the patterns of monosynaptic activation in rat, cat and simian motoneurones. Fig. 1
shows that the stimulating points from which monosynaptic reticulo-motoneuronal actions may be evoked by weak
electrical stimuli (20-100 μa) coincide in the rat, cat
and monkey. A schematic representation of stimulating
sites on the transverse brain stem sections shows that
they are scattered throughout the medial reticular formation, especially in the region of n.reticularis pontis
caudalis, n.reticularis gigantocellularis and fasciculus

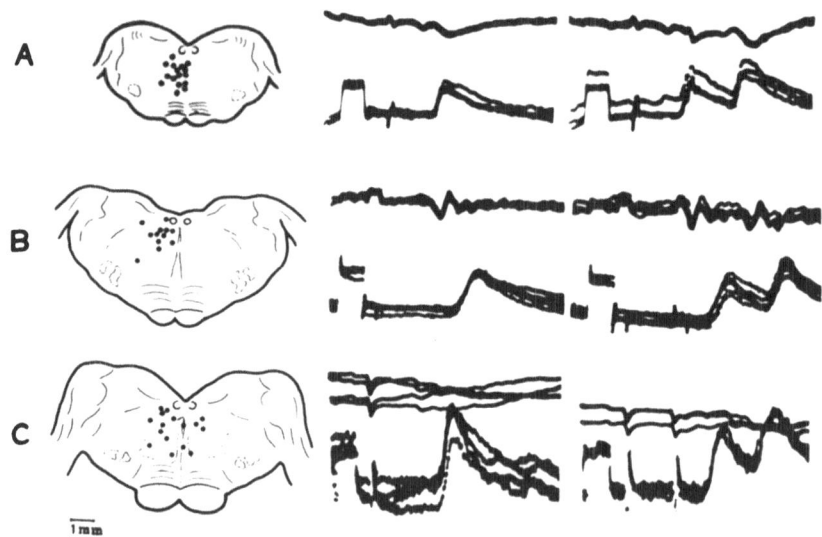

Fig. 1 Comparison of the distribution of points from
        which monosynaptic reticulo-motoneuronal effects
        were evoked and examples of monosynaptic EPSPs
        elicited by single and paired shocks in the rat
        (A), cat (B) and monkey (C). The upper traces
        are records of the cord dorsal potential, the
        lower traces are intracellular records. A calibra-
        tion pulse-2 mv, 1 msec precedes each intracellul-
        ar record (Modified after Shapovalov and Gure-
        vitch, 1970; Shapovalov, 1969; Shapovalov et al.,
        1971)

medialis longitudinalis, i.e. in the same area where
the reticulo-spinal neurones were located by retrograde
degeneration techniques (Brodal, 1957).

The reticulo-motoneuronal EPSPs have a short latency
and are evoked by volleys mediated by the fast-conducting fibers belonging to the fast myelinated fiber group
located in the ventral funiculi. In the rat the conduction velocity of the fastest reticulo-spinal axons reached 70-80 m/sec, in the cat 140-150 m/sec and in the
monkey 80-90 m/sec respectively. All monosynaptic reticulo-motoneuronal EPSPs can be produced by a single
shock and do not show notable growth of amplitude when
the stimuli are repeated. They can follow the stimulating rates up to 500-800 imp/sec and do not sum appreciably until the inter-stimulus interval falls under 3-5
msec. Usually the monosynaptic effects become saturated
by a small increase of the stimulating current and in
some cells the resulting EPSPs ocurred in an all-none
manner, suggesting a strictly limited number of cells
connected with a particular alpha-motoneurone.

In rats and in cats reticulo-spinal volleys monosynaptically excite motoneurones of both proximal and
distal muscle groups, although in cats the maximal
amplitude of reticulo-spinal EPSPs (2,0-2,5 mV) was
found in the motoneurones innervating the proximal
muscles. In the monkey a reticulo-motoneuronal input was
found preferentially in motoneurones of proximal muscles
of the hind-limb.

Stimulation of the same regions of the reticular
formation, from which monosynaptic EPSPs could be elicited, evoked also di- and polysynaptic EPSPs and IPSPs.
Responses with disynaptic segmental delay could be evoked by single shock (Fig. 2) but in many cells detectable
reactions appeared only after repetitive stimulation.
Polysynaptic actions were evoked as a rule only by tetanic stimulation.

In contrast to monosynaptic EPSPs, disynaptic EPSPs
and IPSPs display considerable temporal potentiation
(Fig. 2). This property of potentiation may be of significance in the initiation of a motoneuronal discharge, or
in the case of IPSPs, strongly reinforce the resulting
inhibition. In many cells a single conditioning shock
was followed by an increase of the second response up
to 300-500%.

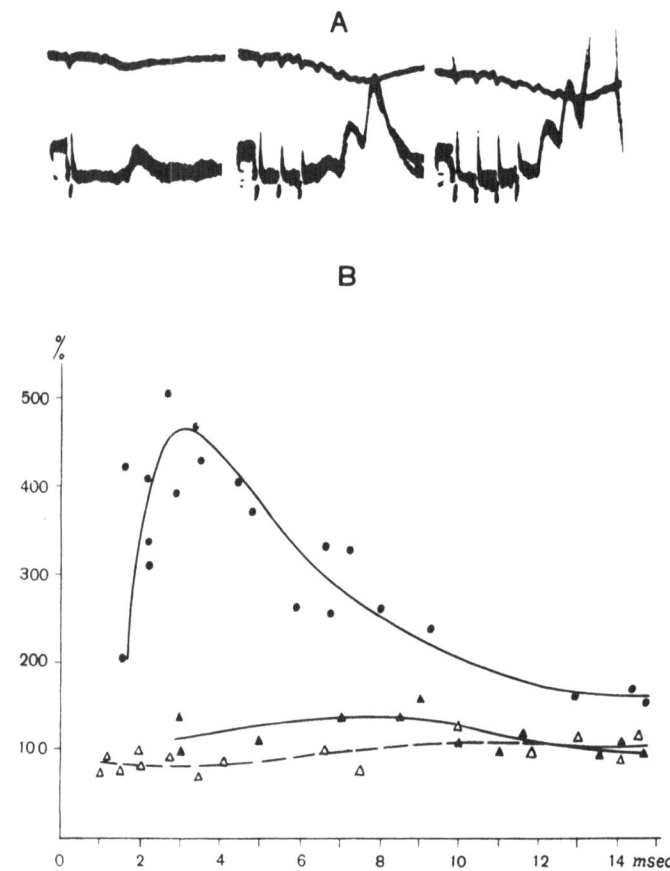

Fig. 2   Properties of disynaptic reticulo-spinal EPSPs.
          A, reticulo-spinal EPSPs evoked in a simian
             motoneurone by single and repetitive volleys.
             Calibration pulse 1 mV, 1 msec.
          B, time-course of potentiation of disynaptic
             (filled cirles) and monosynaptic (triangles)
             EPSPs in a cat motoneurone.Amplitude of EPSPs
             expressed as percent of control amplitude and
             plotted against intervals (in msec.) between
             conditioning and test shocks

     The rubro-spinal pathway connecting the midbrain
with the spinal motor centres develops as the derivative
of the reticulo-spinal system. In the rat and cat rubro-
spinal volleys influence spinal motoneurones presumably
via poly- and disynaptic relays, although in a few individual alpha-motoneurones it was possible to detect
direct rubromotoneuronal input (Shapovalov, 1966; Hongo,
Jankowska and Lundberg, 1969; Gurevitch and Belozerova,

1971). A typical example of disynaptic rubro-spinal
EPSPs potentiated during high-frequency stimulation in
a rat motoneurone is shown in Fig. 3A.

The maximal conduction velocity of the rubro-spinal
fibers in the rat (40-50 m/sec) is considerably smaller
than that typical for the fastest reticulo-spinal fibers
in this species. However, in the cat and monkey there
are practically no differences between the conduction
velocity of the fastest rubro- and reticulo-spinal fibers
respectively.

Experiments carried out on the rhesus monkey (Shapovalov, Karamjan, Kurchavyi and Repina, 1971) showed
that primates possess a considerable monosynaptic projection on the alpha-motoneurones. Monosynaptic rubromotoneuronal EPSPs were evoked by volleys mediated by
fast-conducting fibers, located in the lateral funiculus.
Similar to the reticulo-motoneuronal effects the rubromotoneuronal EPSPs revealed no significant temporal
potentiation and could follow frequencies up to 800 imp/

A

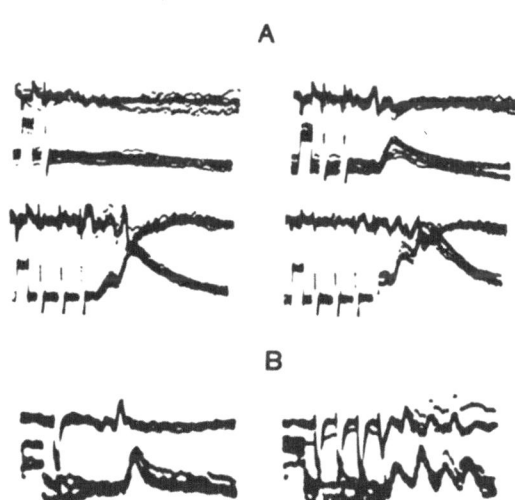

B

Fig. 3   Rubro-spinal effects in the rat (A) and monkey(B).
         A, disynaptic rubro-spinal EPSPs evoked by sing-
            le and repetitive stimuli.Calibration pulse
            2 mV, 1 msec.
         B, monosynaptic rubro-motoneuronal EPSPs evoked
            by single and repetitive stimuli. Calibration
            pulse 1 mV, 1 msec.
         (Modified after Shapovalov et al., 1971)

sec, especially for short periods of stimulation (Fig.3B).

In the monkey the monosynaptic rubro-spinal input
was found mainly in the motoneurones of the distal
muscles of the hind limb (peroneus profundus, extensor
digitorum longus, tibialis anterior, plantaris, flexor
digitorum longus) and shows marked selectivity. Excitatory and inhibitory relations more complex than the
monosynaptic ones exist between the rubro-spinal neurones
and the motoneurones innervating the proximal muscle
groups and m.gastrocnemius.

Evolution of the Deitero-spinal pathway which, as the
rubro-spinal one is derived from the reticular formation
is also characterized by an increase of conduction velocity in comparison with the reticulo-spinal fibers and
by a build up of monosynaptic articulations with spinal
motoneurones (Shapovalov, 1966, 1972 b). Monosynaptic
vestibulo-spinal input is found mostly in the motoneurones of extensor muscles (Grillner, Hongo and Lund,
1970).

Cortical Control of Mammalian Motoneurones

In rodents the cortico-spinal tract is relatively
less developed and less significant in its motor function than in the higher mammals. Recent anatomical
studies indicate that in the rat the pyramidal tract
occupies the most ventral portion of the dorsal column
of white matter and that terminals of cortico-spinal
fibers are distributed only in the dorsal regions of
the dorsal horn subjacent to the substantia gelatinosa
(Brown, 1971). Estimates of the conduction velocities of
the fastest pyramidal tract fibers range from 5 to 15
m/sec (McComas and Wilson, 1966) and thus are 5-10 times
smaller than the maximum conduction velocities of reticulo-spinal fibers in the same species.

We used microstimulation in the depth of the rat
cortex since the effect of intracortical microstimulation is primarily transmitted through the pyramidal
tract (Asanuma and Sakata, 1967). The lowest thresholds
obtained were around 5-10 μa. Upon cortical stimulation
changes in membrane potential were measured in 103
lumbar motoneurones. The responses observed were mostly
depolarizing (90 cells) in a few cases, hyperpolarizing
(9 cells) or complex (3 cells). Practically no effects
were elicited by a single shock. At least a pair of
stimuli was necessary to evoke the minimal detectable

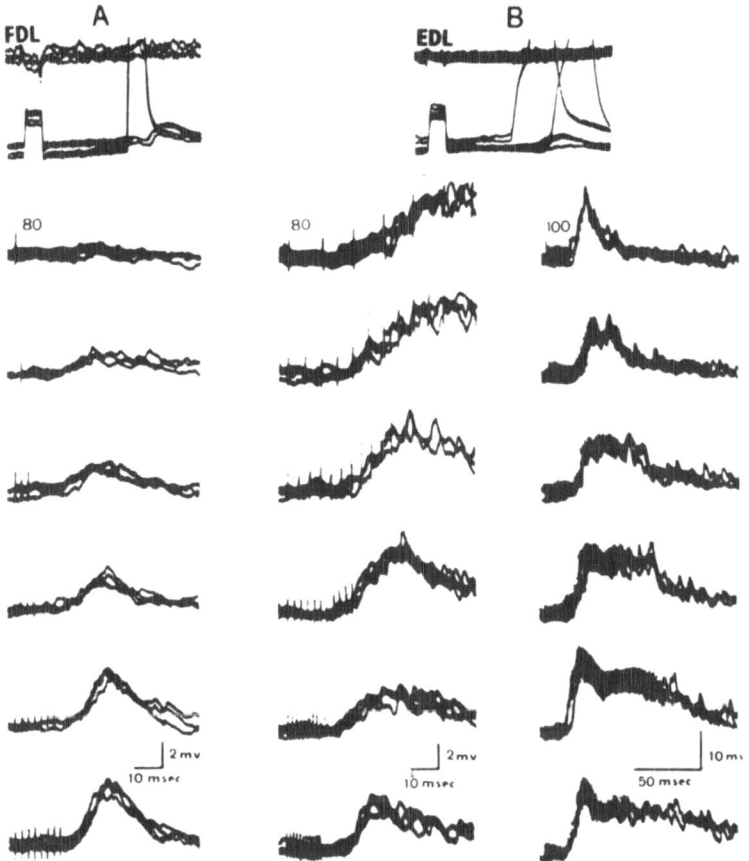

Fig. 4   Effects of intracortical microstimulation in two
         rat motoneurones (A and B).
         A, EPSPs evoked in FDL-motoneurone by single
            and repetitive stimuli
         B, effects evoked in an FDL motoneurone by trains
            of different frequencies (left column) and
            constant frequency but various duration (right
            column). The figures indicate the strength of
            stimulating current (μa). Calibration pulse
            5 mV, 1 msec

EPSP (Fig. 4A). This requirement together with the
minimal latency of the response (10-15 msec) and its
relatively slow rise and complex time course strongly
suggest a polysynaptic linkage. By increasing the number
of applied shocks the depolarization became deeper
until a maximal amplitude (3-4 mV in average) was attained. Cortico-spinal EPSPs only occasionally caused
spike generation. The rate of rise of EPSP increased

with increasing frequency of stimulation (Fig. 4B).
Usually frequencies of 200-300 imp/sec were most effective. A lengthening of the stimulating trains increased
the duration of the post-synaptic response and the depolarization tended to reach a plateau. However, during
long-lasting trains the depolarization decreases even
before the end of cortical stimulation.

    A pyramidal section abolished the cortically in-
duced effects even when much stronger stimulation (up
to 400-500 μa) was used (Fig. 5A). Transection of the
brain stem sparing the bulbar pyramids did not affect
the responses to cortical stimulation (Fig. 5B). These

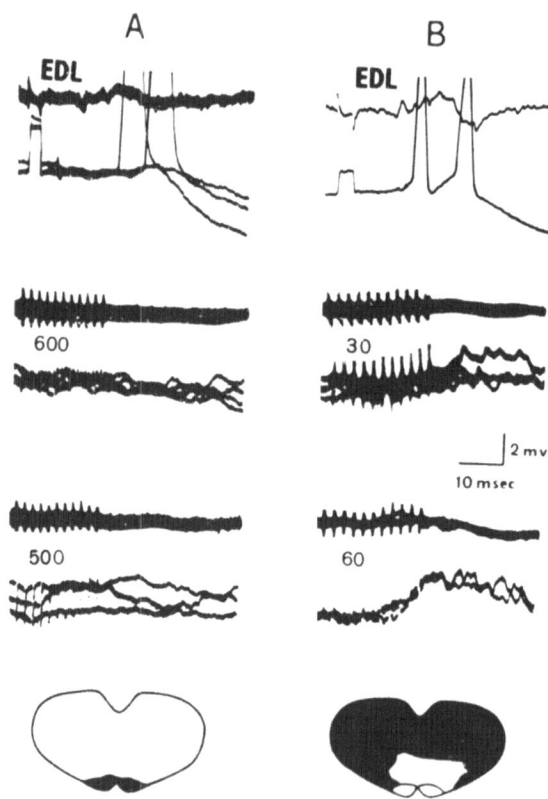

Fig. 5   Effects of intracortical microstimulation in
         rats subjected to pyramidotomy (A) and brain-
         stem section at the medullar level leaving the
         pyramids intact (B).
         Schematic representation of corresponding sec-
         tions is shown below. The figures by each re-
         cord indicate the strength of stimulating cur-
         rent (μA).

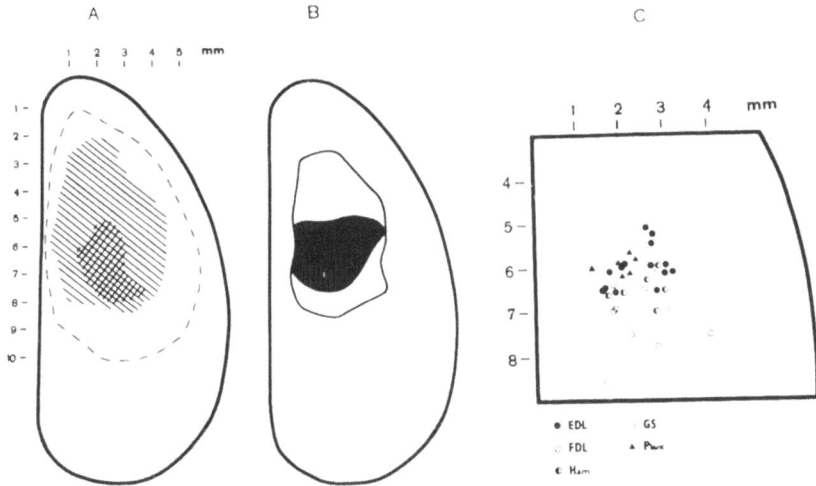

Fig. 6   Diagrams summarizing the location of stimulat-
          ing points on the surface of the rat cortex.
          A, the hatched area shows the region in which
             low-threshold (10-100 µA) spots for evoking
             EPSPs were distributed.
          B, the black area shows the region from which
             contralateral hind-limb movements were evoked
             by intracortical microstimulation.
          C, the distribution of low-threshold spots for
             evoking EPSPs in motoneurones of different
             muscles

results strongly suggest that the pyramidal tract plays
the major role in transmitting this kind of low-threshold cortical effects to the hind-limb motoneurones. Moreover, acute sections of the spinal cord have shown that
the relevant fibers are located in the dorsolateral
funiculi of the spinal cord.

     Systematic mapping of the sites of stimulation re-
vealed that the points with low threshold (10-100 µA)
for evoking EPSPs were concentrated in the same region
from which movements of the hind-limb were produced by
the trains of stimuli (Fig. 6A and B). When the distribution of effective spots within the depth of the cortex
was examined, the most effective depth of stimulation
was found about 200µ and 500-800µ   below the surface
of the cortex, i.e. the histological distribution of
the pyramidal cells is in good correlation with the
location of stimulating electrode (Fig. 7). Droogleever
Fortuyn (1914) reported that this is an agranular area

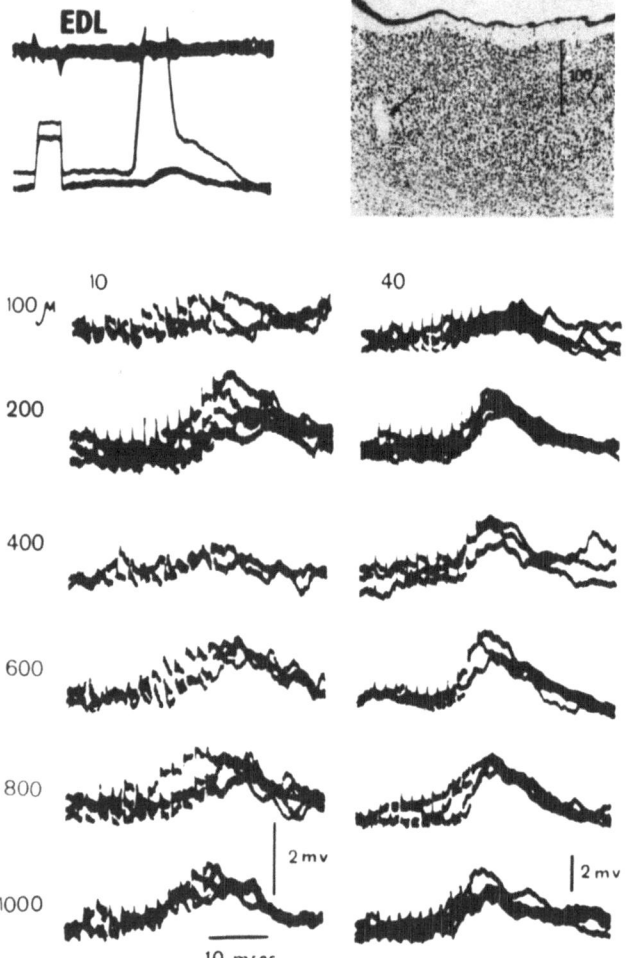

<u>Fig. 7</u> Effects of intracortical microstimulation at
          different depth from the surface on an EDL moto-
          neurone of the rat. The strength of stimulating
          current is 10 μA (left column) and 40 μA(right
          column). The depth of insertion is indicated
          besides each record. The photomicrograph shows
          the position of the stimulating electrode fixed
          at 600 μ

which corresponds to the precentral gyrus in primates.

     Stimulation of the same spots may evoke different
and even opposite effects in different motoneurones.
Intracortical microstimulation evoked EPSPs in the motoneurones of flexors and extensors of distal and proximal

muscle groups. There is a tendency of clustering of the
cortical foci for motoneurones of a particular muscle
in certain regions of the sensori-motor cortex. However,
points of greatest preference for particular motor
nuclei have been found to overlap (Fig. 6 C).

Thus intracortical microstimulation reveals that
in the rat pyramidal effects are exclusively polysynaptic and that there is a marked difference between conduction rates of the fastest pyramidal and reticulo-spinal
projections. Although the amplitudes of the cortico-
spinal and reticulo-spinal effects fall into the same
range of values, the functional role of the former is
small as manifested by ablation experiments (Brown,1971).

In the cat cortico-spinal volleys may activate
spinal motoneurones only via the internuncial neurones
located in the spinal cord (Lloyd, 1941). However, the
conduction velocity of the fastest pyramidal fibers
(about 70 m/sec) is only two times smaller than the conduction velocity of the fastest reticulo-spinal fibers.
Thus, the relative conduction velocity markedly increases in the cat as compared with the rat. The sites
of termination of the cortico-spinal fibers shift more
ventrally and are found in Rexed's lamina VII (Nyberg-
Hansen and Brodal, 1963). Apparently the shortest pathway is disynaptic as the shortest latent period of the
cortico-spinal EPSPs in lumbar motoneurones is 5-6 msec.
Anatomical investigations indicate that in some carnivores (raccoon) terminals of the cortico-spinal fibers
penetrate lamina IX where cell bodies of motoneurones
are located (Buxton and Goodman, 1967).

As the pyramidal system increases in bulk and importance along the phylogenetic range of the mammals it
establishes in primates direct monosynaptic contacts
with spinal alpha-motoneurones (Kuypers, 1960; Phillips,
1969). Single shocks applied to the precentral motor
cortex or bulbar pyramids evoke in the rhesus monkey
pyramidal volleys conducted with a rate of 65-70 m/sec.
This conduction velocity is very near to that typical
for the reticulo-spinal pathway in the same species.
Pyramidal volleys evoke in lumbar motoneurones EPSPs
with monosynaptic segmental delay. Cortico-motoneuronal
EPSPs are in many respects similar to the brain stem-
motoneuronal EPSPs. They are evoked by fast-conducting
fibers and are subthreshold for spike initiation unless
reinforced by background depolarization. However they
have a slower time course and display more marked temporal
potentiation.

A. I. SHAPOVALOV

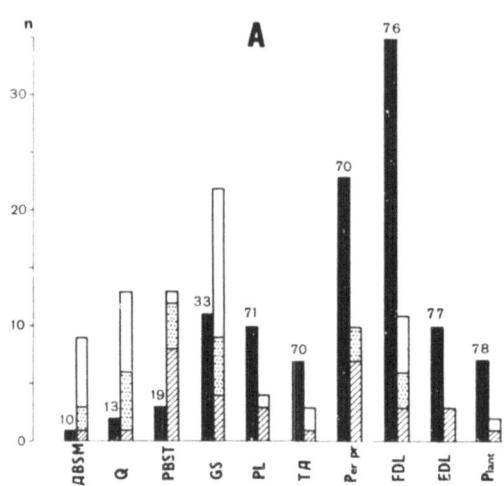

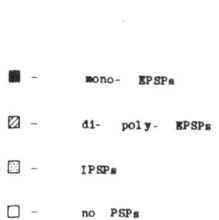

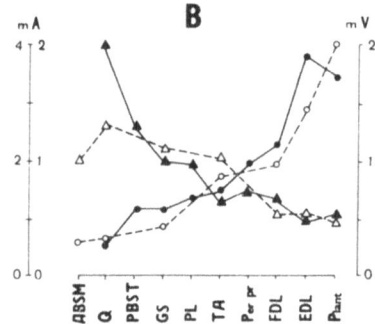

<u>Fig. 8</u>   Cortico-pyramidal effects on motoneurones of
          different muscles in the monkey.
          A, distribution of excitatory and inhibitory
             effects in different motor nuclei. Black
             columns show monosynaptic EPSPs. Ordinate -
             numbers of cells.
          B, average amplitudes of maximal monosynaptic
             EPSPs evoked from motor cortex (filled circles)
             and bulbar pyramids (white circles) and thresh-
             old currents for monosynaptic EPSPs from motor
             cortex (filled triangles) and bulbar pyramids
             (white triangles). Ordinate: right, amplitude
             (mV) left, current: 0-4 mA for the motor
             cortex, 0-2 mA for the bulbar pyramids.

     As was shown by Phillips (1969) on the cervical
motoneurones of the baboon, the largest quantities of
monosynaptic cortico-pyramidal projections are found in
the cells controlling finger movements. Similarly, in
the rhesus monkey monosynaptic cortico-spinal input was

found predominantly in motoneurones innervating the
distal muscles of the hind-limb. Fig. 8 illustrates
that the amplitudes of monosynaptic EPSPs in the motoneurones of the distal muscles are significantly larger
and may be evoked much more frequently than in motoneurones of proximal and gastrocnemius muscles. The
stimulus strength necessary for inducing a monosynaptic
EPSPs was considerably smaller in motoneurones innervating the distal muscles.

The differences between the cortico-pyramidal inputs in these two functional groups of hind-limb motoneurones are not only quantitative. The larger monosynaptic EPSPs in the motoneurones of the distal muscles are
less succeptible to temporal potentiation than the small
EPSPs presumably recorded from motoneurones of the
proximal muscle groups and GS (Fig. 9A). The potentiation of large (1-2 mV) monosynaptic EPSPs usually did
not exceed 130-200% when paired shocks were used, whereas the potentiation of small (0.2 - 0.5 mV) EPSPs could
attain 300-500% under similar conditions as in the case

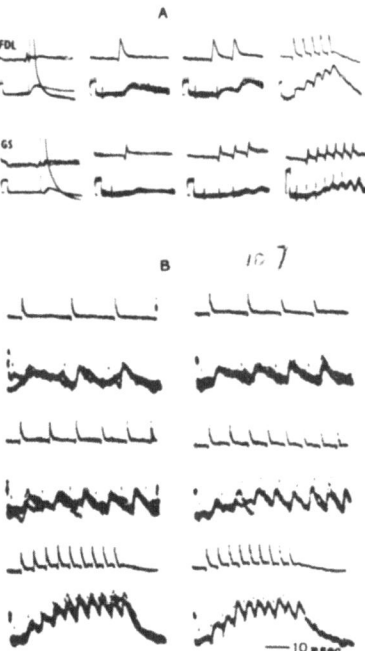

Fig. 9 Monosynaptic EPSPs evoked in different simian
        motoneurones from the motor cortex (A) and
        bulbar pyramids (B).
        A, calibration pulse 5 mV, 1 msec for FDL and
          GS, 2 mV, 1 msec for all other records.
        B, calibration pulse 2 mV

of disynaptic EPSPs. Direct stimulation of the bulbar
pyramids when an activation of intracortical circuits
is prevented, also reveals only a moderate temporal
potentiation (Fig. 9B).

    In monkeys with pyramidal section there was a com-
plete abolition of the direct pyramidal volleys and of
the monosynaptic cortico-motoneuronal EPSPs. However,
motoneurones receiving strong monosynaptic input as
evidenced by their responses to bulbar pyramidal stimulation, could be also activated by repetitive stimulation
of the motor cortex (Fig. 10). The latency of cortico-
extrapyramidal EPSPs was over 8-10 msec. The pattern
of synaptic activation tended to be diffuse, i.e. not
time-locked with the applied shocks. Obviously the poly-

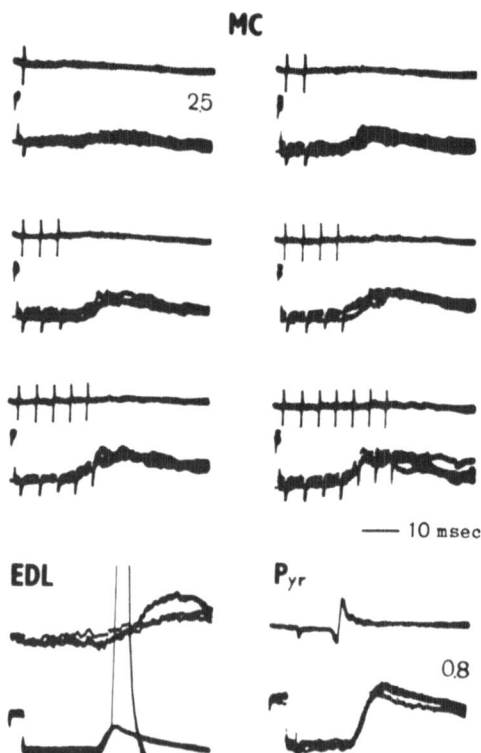

Fig. 10 Cortico-extrapyramidal effects in a pyramido-
         tomised monkey. Effects evoked by single and re-
         petitive stimulation of motor cortex(MC) at in-
         tensity 2.5 mA and single shock applied to
         bulbar pyramid (Pyr). Calibration pulse 2 mV,
         for MC; 2 mV, 1 msec for Pyr; 5 mV, 1 msec for
         FDL.

synaptic cortico-extrapyramidal projections are far less
efficient than the direct cortico-pyramidal pathways
which is consistent with the severe motor deficit induced by pyramidal section.

CONCLUSIONS

The present data indicate that the fast reticulo-
spinal fibers build monosynaptic connections with spinal motoneurones in all mammals, even in a species at a
relatively low stage of encephalization, and that the
differences between direct reticulo-motoneuronal projections in different mammalian species are mainly
quantitative and not qualitative. Evidently, in the
course of evolution the efficient reticulo-motoneuronal
projection was developed at an early stage (cf.Shapova-
lov, 1972 b) and was very little changed thereafter. It
may be suggested that it plays as important role in
motor coordination otherwise it would not have been preserved throughout all the evolution range.

The development of younger supraspinal systems:
vestibulo-, rubro- and cortico-spinal is characterized
by the increase of conduction rate of relevant descending pathways in comparison with the fast reticulo-spinal
fibers and by a development of direct monosynaptic
articulations with particular alpha-motoneurones. Thus
direct cerebro-motoneuronal linkage is not a unique
feature of any brain level. Whatever the exact nature of
the supraspinal organization the present results suggest
that the basic design of cerebro-spinal projection includes colonies of large fast-conducting neurones directly connected with particular alpha-motoneurones.

At present there is no conclusive evidence about
the exact functional significance of direct descending
projections. It may be suggested that an interpretation
of their role should be based on the following facts:
1) monosynaptic effects are fast, 2) they may be accomp-
lished by a relatively small number of cells and need
far less energy in order to reach the same effect as
ordinary sustained depolarization (cf. Shapovalov, 1972a);
3) monosynaptic commands supply the motoneurones with
information whose processing has been completed at the
brain level and which is not distorted at the spinal
levels; 4) monosynaptic commands may be more specific
in terms of selective activation of particular functional groups of motoneurones; 5) the simple direct circuits

may be more effectively subserved by internal feed-back mechanisms. These features may be particularly advantageous as compared with more diffuse polysynaptic projections and this advantage may account for the preservation of this design pattern from the most primitive to the most evolved mammals, from the oldest to the newest levels of the brain.

The role of the more abundant polysynaptic projections is also far from certain. Apparently an efficient supraspinal control requires a cooperation between specific and diffuse projections, of pyramidal and extrapyramidal influences. In fact, the monosynaptic actions usually can affect the patterning of motoneuronal discharges only when combined with polysynaptic reinforcement. As Granit (1970) has pointed out, a non-specific effect may be all that is needed for eliciting a specific effect, providing a kind of necessary background of general depolarization for the commands mediated by the direct inputs.

REFERENCES

ASANUMA H. & SAKATA H. (1967). Functional organization of a cortical efferent system examined with focal depth stimulation in cats. J.Neurophysiol., 30: 35-54.

BOGATYREVA E.S. & SHAPOVALOV A. I. (1973). Synaptic actions evoked by intracortical microstimulation in lumbar motoneurones of the rat. Neurofisiologie (Kiev), in press.

BRODAL A. (1957). The reticular formation of the brain stem. Edinburgh: Oliver & Boyd.

BROWN L. T. (1971). Projections and termination of the corticospinal tract in rodents. Exper.Brain Res., 13: 432-450.

BUXTON D. F. & GOODMAN D. C. (1967). Motor function and the corticospinal tracts in the dog and raccoon. J. Comp.Neurol., 129: 341-360.

DROOGLEEVER FORTUYN A. B. (1914). Cortical cell-lamination of the hemispheres of some rodents. Arch.Neurol. Psychiat., 6: 221-354.

GRANIT R. (1970). The Basis of Motor Control. London, Academic Press.

GRILLNER S., HONGO T. & LUND S. (1970). The vestibulo-spinal tract. Effects of alpha-motoneurones in the lumbosacral spinal cord in the cat. Exper.Brain Res., 10: 94-120.

GUREVITCH N. R. & BELOZEROVA T. V. (1971). Rubrospinal synaptic influences on lumbar motoneurones in the rat. Neurofisiologia (Kiev), 3: 274-284.

HONGO T., JANKOWSKA E. & LUNDBERG A. (1969). The rubro-
spinal tract. I. Effects on alpha-motoneurones innervating hind-limb muscles in cats. Exp.Brain Res., 7: 344-
364.
KUYPERS H. G. J. M. (1960). Central cortical projections
to the motor and somato-sensory cell groups. An experimental study in Rhesus monkey. Brain. 83: 161-184.
LLOYD D. P. C. (1941). The spinal mechanism of the
pyramidal system in cats. J.Neurophysiol., 4: 525-540.
McCOMAS A. J. & WILSON P. (1966). Some properties of
pyramidal tract cells in the rat somatosensory cortex.
J.Physiol.(Lond.),I88: 35-36 p.
NYBERG-HANSEN R. & BRODAL A. (1963). Sites of termination of cortico-spinal fibers in the cat. An experimental study with silver impregnation methods. J.Comp.
Neurol., 120: 369-391.
PHILLIPS C. G. (1969). Motor apparatus of the baboon's
hand. Proc.Roy.Soc.B. 173: 141-174.
TAMAROVA Z. A., SHAPOVALOV A. I., KARAMJAN O. A. & KUR-
CHAVYI G. G. (1972). Cortico-pyramidal and cortico-
extrapyramidal synaptic actions on lumbar motoneurones
in the monkey. Neurofisiologia (Kiev), 4 (in press).
SHAPOVALOV A. I. (1966). Excitation and inhibition of
spinal neurones during supraspinal stimulation. In:
Nobel Symposium I.,ed.Granit R., pp. 331-348. Stockholm: Almqvist & Wiksell.
SHAPOVALOV A. I. (1969). Post-tetatic potentiation of
monosynaptic and disynaptic actions from supraspinal
structures on lumbar motoneurones. J.Neurophysiol.,
32: 325-348.
SHAPOVALOV A. I. (1972 a). Extrapyramidal monosynaptic
and disynaptic control of mammalian alpha-motoneurones.
Brain Research. 40: 105-115.
SHAPOVALOV A. I. (1972 b). Evolution of neuronal systems
of supraspinal motor control. Neurophysiologia (Kiev),
4, in press.
SHAPOVALOV A. I. & GUREVITCH N. R. (1970). Monosynaptic
and disynaptic reticulospinal actions on lumbar motoneurones of the rat. Brain Research. 21: 249-263.
SHAPOVALOV A. I., KARAMYAN O. A., KURCHAVYI G. G. & RE-
PINA Z. A. (1971). Synaptic actions evoked from the
red nucleus on the spinal alpha-motoneurones in the
Rhesus monkey. Brain Research. 32: 325-348.
SHAPOVALOV A. I., KURCHAVYI G. G., KARAMYAN O. A. & RE-
PINA Z. A. (1971). Extrapyramidal pathways with mono-
synaptic effects upon primate alpha-motoneurones.
Experientia (Basel). 27: 522-524.

SUPRASPINAL MECHANISMS OF MOTOR CONTROL

P. G. KOSTYUK

From the S.S.Bogomoletz Institute of Physiology

Kiev, USSR

The control of spinal reflex mechanisms from supraspinal structures is exerted in the most developed form
(in mammals) by four descending systems (cortico-, rubro-,
reticulo- and vestibulo-spinal). Other descending systems
(for instance, tecto- and interstitio-spinal) being obviously quite important in the early stages of the evolu-
tionary development of the vertebrate nervous system
have become in mammals of secondary importance comparing
to the above-mentioned systems. Probably because of that
they usually remain outside the field of morphological
and electrophysiological investigations. All these systems are tightly functionally interconnected during
natural reflex activity, and it is usually very difficult
to separate the contribution of each of them to the
mechanism of the motor act. Nevertheless using an analyt-
ical approach it is still possible to define certain
specific features in the activity of each descending
system.

It is well known that the descending systems can
be grouped according to certain principles. Probably
their division into lateral (cortico- and rubro-spinal)
and medial (vestibulo- and reticulo-spinal) systems as
proposed by Kuypers (1964) is in best accordance with
the presence of intersystemic relations and common in-
trinzic properties. The lateral systems are characterized by location of their descending fibers in the
dorsolateral funiculus. Their terminals have predominant
connection with the interneuronal apparatus of the

lateral part of the base of the dorsal horn, which in turn
is projected to the lateral motor nuclei. Being phylogenetically young these systems are well developed only
in mammals. The vestibulo- and reticulo-spinal descending systems which form the medial systems are characterized by a common location in the ventral funiculus and
similar modes of termination on the ventro-medial segmental neuronal apparatus. They both are phylogenetically
old systems and are well developed in all classes of
vertebrates.

LATERAL SYSTEMS

Structurally the lateral systems are prominent by
the presence of exact somatotopic organization of their
projections; at the same time they contain (especially
the cortico-spinal system) predominantly thin, slowly-
conducting fibers which do not establish direct connections to motoneurones. Only in primates (and also in a
few other mammals capable to produce fine movements of
the digits) a limited number of cortico-spinal fibers
does reach the motoneurones. Therefore it is natural to
suggest that the spinal interneuronal apparatus must
play a very important role in the realization of the
commands coming through the lateral systems. Such commands govern mainly fast flexor movements of different
parts of the limbs.

The location of interneurones primarily related to
the lateral descending systems is now precisely determih-
ed by both morphological and electrophysiological
methods. In experimental morphological studies the location of degenerating preterminals of these systems was
traced by the techniques of Nauta (Nyberg-Hansen and
Brodal, 1963, 1964) and Fink-Heimer, Kostyuk, Pogorelaya
and Dyachkova, 1972; Kostyuk and Skibo, 1972b); in the
latter investigations the location of corresponding
synaptic terminals was determined also electron-micro-
scopically. In electrophysiological studies the spatial
distribution of extracellular field potentials was
measured at short intervals after the arrival of a descending volley in the spinal gray matter (Lloyd, 1941;
Vasilenko and Kostyuk, 1965; Pilyavsky and Skibo, 1969;
Bayev and Kostyuk, 1972 a,b). All these studies gave
comparable results: cat's interneurones primarily connected to the cortico-spinal fibers are located in the
lateral part of Rexed's laminae IV-VI, and those primarily connected to rubro-spinal fibers, in the lateral
parts of laminae VI-VII. There is a certain overlap be-

tween these areas; a small number of terminals reaches
also other interneuronal groups.

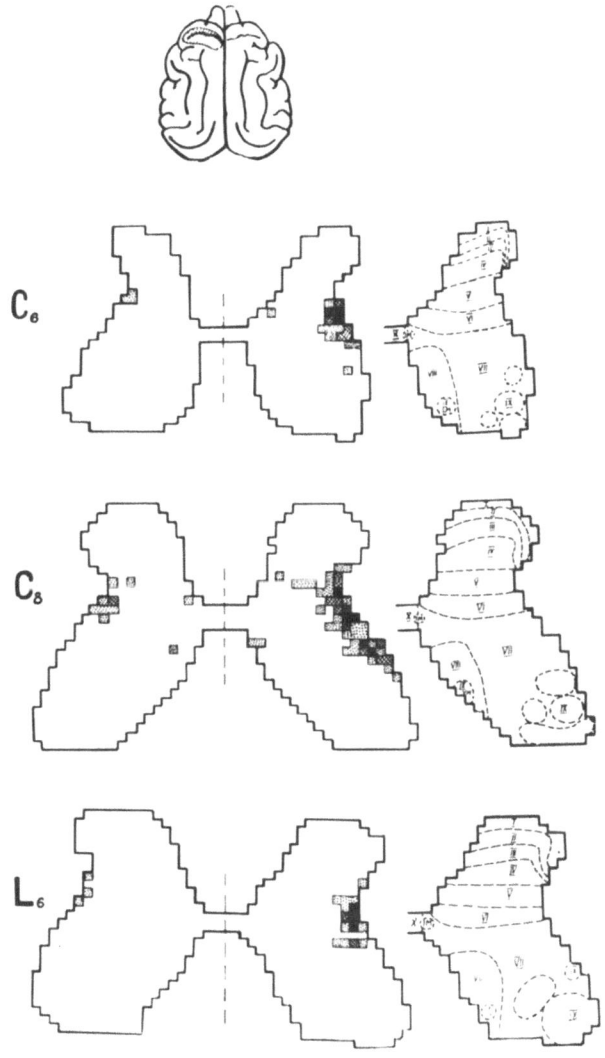

Fig. 1   Quantitative distribution of cortico-spinal pre-
          terminal fibers in cross-sections of different
          spinal segments in the cat. The destroyed region
          of the cortex is shown at the top. The number of
          degenerated preterminals was calculated in
          squares 100μ x 100μ. Dotted squares indicate
          5-10 degenerating fragments, hatched: 10-15 and
          filled: over 15. Italics on the right schemes de-
          note the Rexed's laminae (Kostyuk, Pogorelaya
          and Dyachkova, 1972).

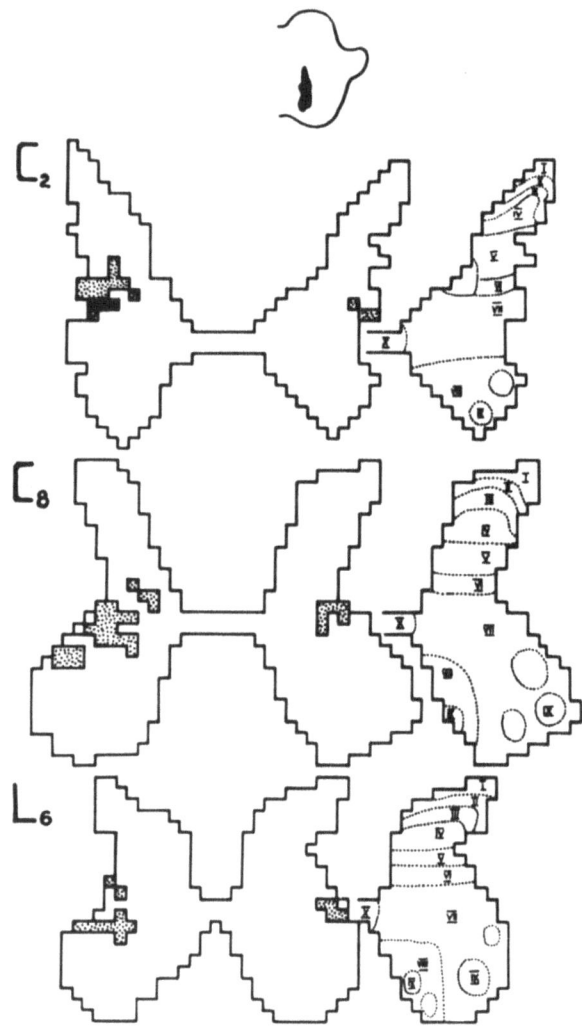

Fig. 2   Quantitative distribution of rubro-spinal pre-
         terminal fibers in cross-sections of different
         spinal segments in the cat. The destroyed re-
         gion of the midbrain is shown above. The schemes
         are constructed as in Fig. 1.

         Fig. 1 and 2 present maps showing the quantitative
distribution of cortico- and rubro-spinal preterminals
in different segments of the cat spinal cord as determined by the Fink-Heimer technique.

         The microelectrode recording of responses of
single cell in the indicated areas shows that many of
them can be antidromically excited by stimulation of

the dorso-lateral funiculus in more caudally located
segments. Therefore these cells may be classified as
propriospinal neurones (Vasilenko, Zadorozhny and

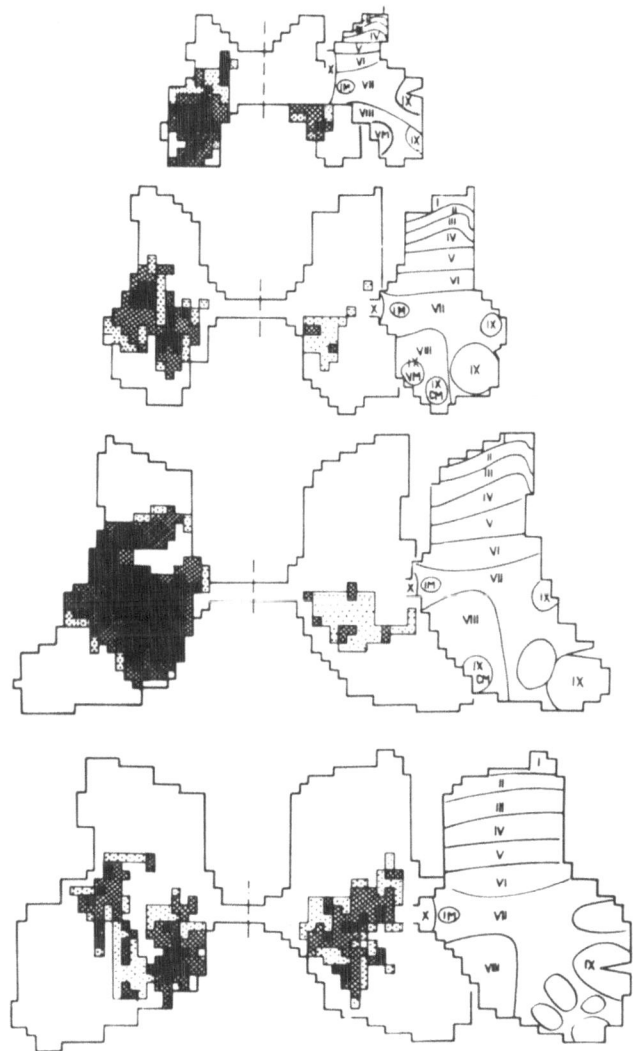

Fig. 3   Quantitative distribution of propriospinal pre-
         terminal fibers from the lateral funiculus in
         cross-sections of different lumbar segments of the
         spinal cord of the cat.The lateral funiculus was
         destroyed at the 3rd lumbar segment.A preliminary
         section of long descending pathways was made at
         the first lumbar segment. Dotted squares indicate
         5-10 degenerating fragments, hatched: 10-15 and
         filled:over 15 (Kostyuk and Maisky, 1972).

Kostyuk, 1967). Morphological investigations carried out using the method of double sections of the spinal cord separated in time have also shown that the proprio-spinal axons in the lateral funiculus originate from neurones in this region; they extend over a distance of up to 4 segments and terminate both in the dorso-lateral motor nuclei and in the intermediate gray matter (Kostyuk and Maisky, 1972; see Fig.3).

Such propriospinal neurones are always effectively synaptically activated by the cortico- and rubro-spinal systems, and sometimes also by fast reticulo-spinal pathways. The relative effectiveness of synaptic influences can be different in different cells: in some of them (usually those located more dorsally) the cortico-spinal volley is more effective, in others (those located more ventrally), it is the rubro-spinal volley. Equal effects are also possible. Judging from the value of the

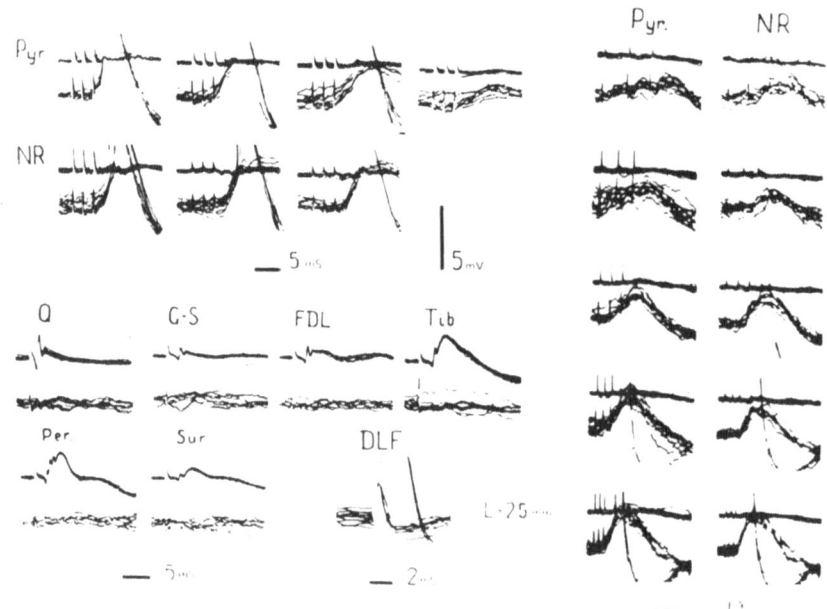

Fig. 4   Intracellularly recorded responses of a proprio-spinal neurone to stimulation of the medullary pyramids (Pyr) and red nucleus (NR). The 3-shock stimulation was changed in strength (upper left records) and frequency (right records). The absence of synaptic responses to a 10 times threshold strong stimulation of peripheral nerves and antidromic activation from the dorso-lateral funiculus (DLF) are also shown (lower left records)(Vasilenko,Kostyukov and Pilyavsky, 1972).

segmental synaptic delay in a considerable number of recorded neurones the descending effects should be monosynaptic (Bayev and Kostyuk, 1972 a,b;Vasilenko, Kostyukov and Pilyavsky, 1972).

At the same time, here the synaptic effects from
peripheral afferents are late and weak, in many cells
they altogether cannot be revealed even after stimulation of the whole dorsal funiculus (that means after un-
dubitable stimulation of all peripheral inputs to the
cord). An example of intracellular recording illustrat-
ing these properties of a propriospinal neurone is shown
on Fig. 4.

The propriospinal neurones in the dorso-lateral

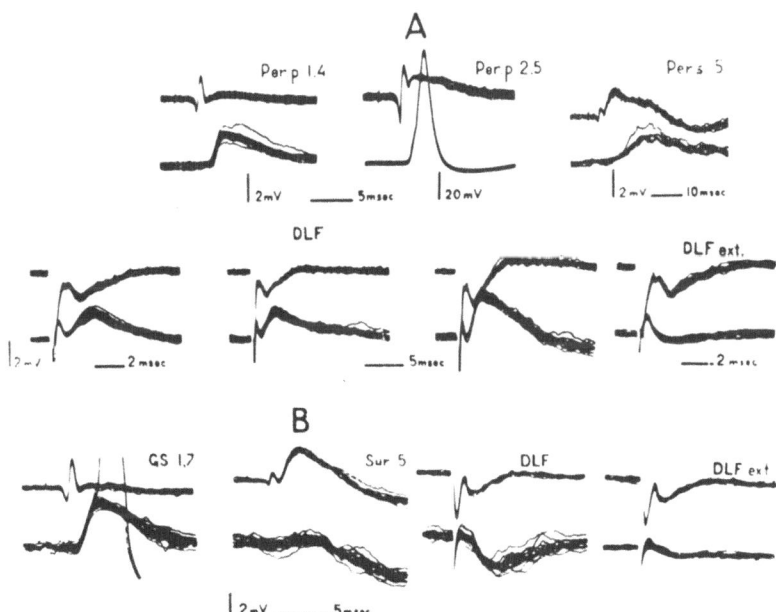

Fig. 5   Examples of postsynaptic potentials evoked in
         flexor (A) and extensor (B) motoneurones by a
         stimulation of propriospinal fibers in the
         dorso-lateral funiculus. Responses to peripheral
         nerve stimulation are also shown. Strength of
         stimuli is given as multiples of the threshold.
         The third oscillogram in the lower row of A was
         obtained with increased strength of DLF stimula-
         tion. The last oscillograms in A and B (DLF ext)
         were recorded extracellularly just outside the
         cell (Kostyuk, Vasilenko and Lang, 1971).

funiculus can probably transmit their activity directly
to the motoneurones. This is confirmed by the observation that a separate stimulation of the propriospinal
fibers(produced in animals with preliminary sectioned
funiculi so that long descending pathways are degenerated and only the propriospinal ones remain excitable)
can produce in the motoneurones monosynaptic responses
similar to those produced by activation of the lateral
descending systems (Kostyuk, Vasilenko and Lang, 1971).
Oscillograms showing such effects are presented on
Fig. 5.

In this way the motor signals reaching the spinal
cord through the lateral descending systems may be integrated to a considerable extent in the propriospinal
interneuronal apparatus, and the motoneurones do not
receive information about the way they reach the cord.
This is probably reflected in the extreme similarity of
pyramidal and rubral effects at motoneurones. At the
same time the possibility of transmission of specialized
descending commands to motoneurones cannot be ruled out
completely.

It must be noted that the propriospinal neurones
with axons passing through the dorso-lateral funiculus

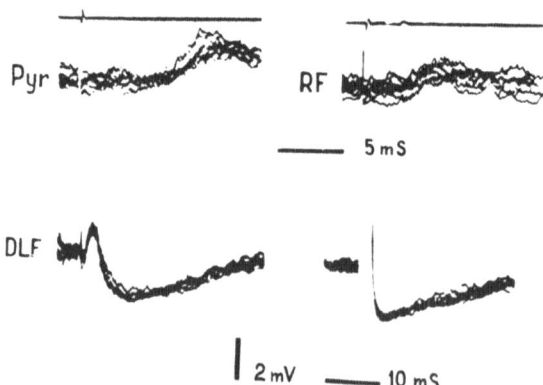

Fig. 6   Intracellularly recorded responses of a proprio-
          spinal neurone of the dorso-lateral funiculus
          to a stimulation of the medullar pyramids (Pyr),
          medial reticular formation(RF) and dorso-lateral
          funiculus(DLF).In tha latter case the stimulus
          strength was subthreshold (left) and suprathresh-
          old (right) for the antidromic excitation of
          the cell (Vasilenko, Kostyukov and Anastasije-
          vić, unpublished).

possess certain functional properties which can influence
the motor signal transmitted through them. First, the
generation of action potentials here is followed by
strong after-hyperpolarization combined with IPSP of unknown origin that eliminate all preexisting synaptic
processes (Fig. 6). Therefore such neurones cannot
generate a long-lasting high-frequency discharge. Even
during high-frequency stimulation of the motor cortex or
the red nucleus their discharge is limited to a level
below 50 imp./sec. Second, the postsynaptic responses
produced by propriospinal volleys in motoneurones are
easily potentiated. They sharply differ in this respect
from monosynaptic responses produced in the same cells
by group Ia afferent volleys (Fig. 7). Probably such
properties facilitate the transmission of signals in
form of bursts to the motoneurones and at the same time
hinder background rhythmic activity.

The situation is different in the interneurones of
the intermediate gray matter which are easily activated
by primary afferents and from the segmental interneuronal

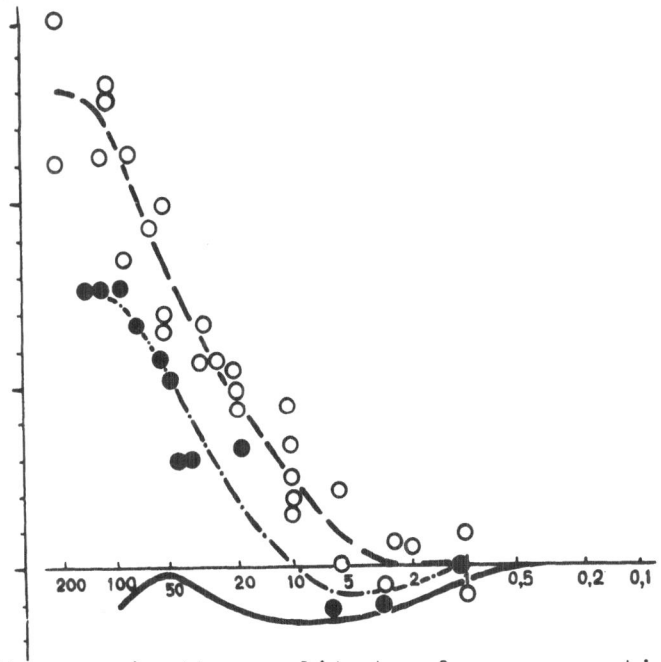

Fig. 7   Changes in the amplitude of monosynaptic EPSP
          and IPSP in motoneurones with variations in the
          frequency of stimulation of propriospinal fibers
          (DLF) and group Ia afferents. Abscissa: stimulation
          frequency, ordinate: relative PSP amplitude (PSP
          amplitude during stimulation once every 2 seconds
          is taken as unity).

apparatus. Such neurones are also subjected to influences from the lateral systems, resulting in development of EPSP and facilitating the polysynaptic reflex
responses in the motoneurones. However, this action is
always delayed and mediated through some other interneurones - perhaps through the propriospinal ones (Lundberg, Norrsell and Voorhoeve, 1962).

As in this case the interneurones are shared by
both descending and segmental mechanisms, one may suggest that their functional role might change corresponding to the relative effectiveness of converging descending and peripheral synaptic influences. During
strong afferent and subthreshold descending volleys the

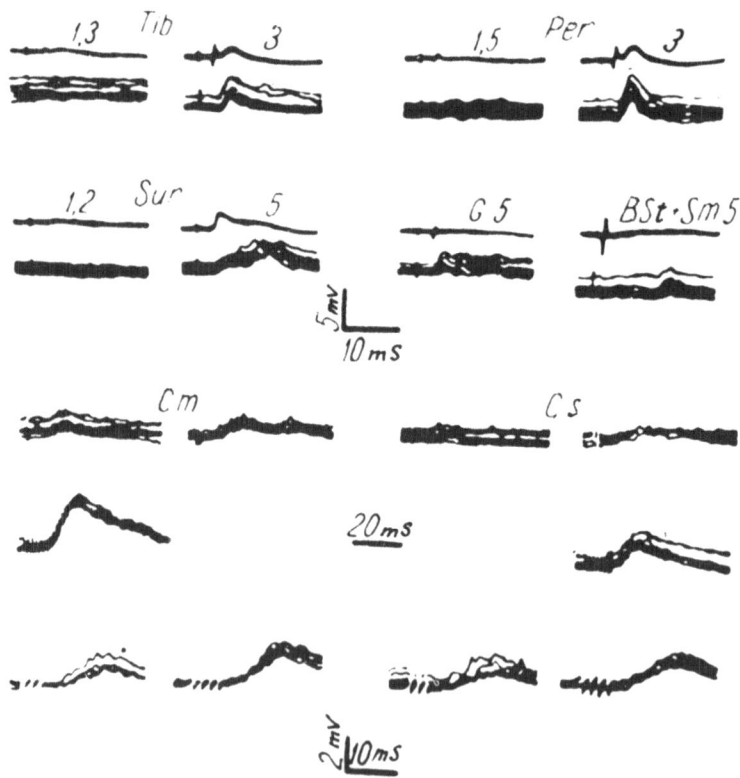

Fig. 8   Corticofugal influences from the somatosensory
          (Cs) and motor areas (Cm) upon an interneurone
          activated by flexor reflex afferents. The
          strength of peripheral nerve stimulation is in-
          dicated as multiples of threshold (Zadorozhny,
          Vasilenko and Kostyuk, 1970).

latter will have mainly a modulating function, facilitating (or releasing) the activity of certain spinal mechanisms. During opposite relations the same neurones may serve as transmitters of commands coming from the brain, and the peripheral influences may be of secondary importance.

Considering the action of the lateral descending systems upon segmentary interneurones it should be noticed that this action is particularly effective in the interneurones connected to high-threshold peripheral afferents (so called flexor reflex afferents). In these neurones descending volleys produce very strong EPSP's which often are by themselves sufficient to generate a neuronal discharge (Zadorozhny, Vasilenko and Kostyuk, 1970). An example of these EPSP's is shown on Fig. 8. Strongly facilitated are also all final effects produced by such afferent volleys in motoneurones and neurones of the ascending pathways (e.g., IPSP in dorsal-spino- cerebellar tract neurones).

Obviously it would be an oversimplification to consider the interneuronal system connected to high-threshold cutaneous and muscle afferents as serving only for the generation of a defensive flexor reflex. In certain conditions this system can take part in much more complicated motor reactions programmed by spinal neuronal structures (e.g., in locomotion). Its facilitation from the lateral descending systems probably reveals a component of the suprasegmental control mechanism governing such reactions. Elucidation of this question could be achieved only by using more specific ways of activation of the corresponding interneurones.

Finally- the descending signals coming through the lateral systems exert a marked influence upon the central afferent terminals, producing a long-lasting depolarization (Carpenter, Lundberg and Norrsell, 1963; Andersen, Eccles and Sears, 1964). This action is also directed mainly to terminals of high-threshold fibers, it is absent in group Ia fibers. Because of the presynaptic depolarization of high-threshold fibers, the effectiveness of the synaptic action of impulses coming through them should be decreased; perhaps such a limitation of the afferent inflow is one of the mechanisms switching the interneuronal system to the fulfilment of other tasks.

MEDIAL SYSTEMS

Structurally the medial systems have fibers of
large diameter with very high conduction velocity. Morphological studies performed both by detection of degenerating preterminal elements (Nyberg-Hansen, 1966) and by
electron-microscopic investigation of degenerating
synaptic endings (Kostyuk and Skibo, 1972a) indicate
that these fibers are primarily connected to neurones
of the intermediate gray matter and the medial part of
the ventral horn (laminae VII-VIII according to Rexed).
Here they establish synaptic connections not only with
interneurones but also with motoneurones (through their
dendrites extending into the dorsomedial part of the
ventral horn). Despite this, the somatotopic organization is less pronounced in the medial systems comparing to the lateral ones and their synaptic effects are
much more diffuse, extending over large neuronal popula-
tions. A scheme of the location of preterminal elements
of the medial systems in different segments of the
spinal cord of the cat is shown on Fig.9.

Among the medial systems the medial reticulo-spinal and lateral vestibulo-spinal tracts are the best defined morphologically and functionally. The medial
reticulo-spinal tract originates from the medial reticular structures of the brain stem (n.reticularis
pontis oralis et caudalis, part of n.gigantocellularis).
Its fibers pass in the medial part of the ventral funiculus mainly homolaterally and have conduction velocity
up to 130 m/sec. They reach the most caudal segments of
the spinal cord. The lateral vestibulo-spinal tract
begins from neurones of the lateral (Deiters) vestibular
nucleus and descends in the lateral part of the ventral
funiculus down to the caudal lumbar segments.

At the same time, a large number of reticulo-spinal fibers having lower conduction velocity originate
from more lateral reticular structures of the medulla
and descend bilaterally in the lateral parts of the
ventral funiculi (the lateral reticulo-spinal tracts).
A part of the vestibulo-spinal fibers coming from the
medial vestibular nucleus (and also from the ventral
portion of the Deiters' nucleus) converge near the mid-
line and descend in the spinal cord in the form of the
medial vestibulo-spinal tract. They can be traced down
only to the thoracic segments. It must be noted that

the ventral funiculi contain also a considerable amount
of propriospinal pathways which can be synaptically connected to the descending systems; this makes their analysis much more difficult.

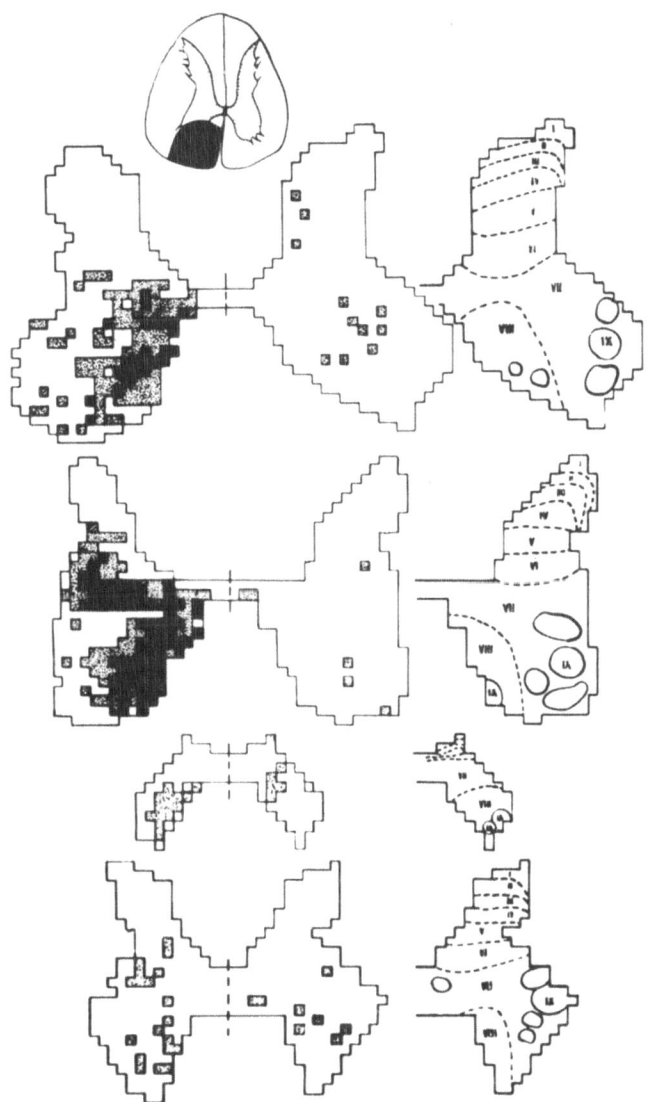

Fig. 9   Quantitative distribution of preterminals of the
         medial descending systems in cross-sections of
         different spinal segments in the cat. Unilateral
         section of the ventral funiculus was performed
         at the level of first cervical segment (as in-
         dicated above). The schemes are constructed as
         in Fig. 3 (Kostyuk and Skibo, 1972).

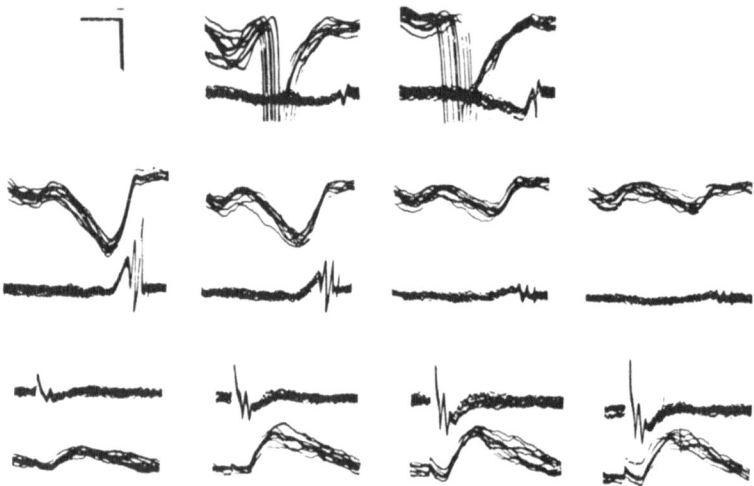

Fig. 10   Monosynaptic EPSP in a thoracic motoneurone of
          the spinal cord of the cat produced by stimula-
          tion of the medial part of n.gigantocellularis
          (RF) and ventral funiculus (FV). The strength
          of stimulation is indicated as multiples of
          threshold (Preobrazhensky, Bezhenaru and Gokin,
          1969).

The effects produced in spinal motoneurones by the
fast-conducting fibers of the medial reticulo-spinal and
lateral vestibulo-spinal tracts can be distinguished
very precisely. Lund and Pompeiano (1965) were the first
to show that stimulation of the ventral funiculus at the
thoracic level produces monosynaptic EPSP's both in extensor and flexor lumbar motoneurones. If the Deiters'
nucleus was preliminary destroyed so that the vestibulo-
spinal fibers degenerated, the same stimulation failed
to produce monosynaptic EPSP's in extensor motoneurones
but they still could be elicited in flexor motoneurones.
It is clear that monosynaptic EPSP's in extensor motoneurones in such experiments are of vestibular origin
and those in flexor motoneurones - of nonvestibular. As
similar monosynaptic EPSP's in flexor cells could be
evoked by stimulation of the medial reticular formation,
it was concluded that they are produced by reticulo-
spinal fibers (Grillner and Lund, 1966; 1968; Shapovalov,
Grantyn and Kurchavyi, 1967). The conduction velocity

in the corresponding reticulo-spinal fibers is 100-
150 m/sec. Direct stimulation of the Deiters' nucleus
also produces monosynaptic EPSP's in extensor motoneurones (Shapovalov, Kurchavyi and Strogonova, 1966).

Monosynaptic EPSP of reticular origin can be regularly detected in thoracic motoneurones (Preobrazhensky, Bezhenaru and Gokin, 1969) and in motoneurones of
upper cervical segments. In the latter case, contrary
to lumbar segments, monosynaptic EPSP produced by
stimulation of both reticular formation and vestibular
nuclei can be observed in the same cells. Such motoneurones probably innervate nuclei not belonging to any
of the antagonist groups: flexors or extensors, and
produce movements of the head (Wilson and Yoshida,
1969a,b). Fig. 10 presents examples of reticular monosynaptic EPSP in cat thoracic motoneurones.

It is natural to suggest that the direct contacts
of fast-conducting fibers of the medial systems to motoneurones represent only a minor part of their terminals,
and that most of them are terminating on interneurones
in the medial part of the ventral horn, therefore such
fibers should also induce considerable polysynaptic effects upon motoneurones. In fact, monosynaptic responses
in motoneurones are regularly followed by delayed responses, especially after a certain increase of intensity of stimulation. Correspondingly some direct synaptic effects produced by reticulo- and vestibulo-spinal
volleys can be recorded from single interneurones. Thus,
in many interneurones related to the muscle afferents
of the group I, monosynaptic EPSP's are produced via
fast-conducting reticulo-spinal pathways (see example
on Fig.11). Such EPSP's were observed also in some cells
which could not be activated by peripheral afferents.
At the same time, interneurones connected to the low
threshold cutaneous afferents and to the interneurones
that have synaptic inputs only from high-threshold afferents did not respond to such a descending volley or
showed late irregular responses (Bezhenaru, Gokin, Zadorozhny and Preobrazhensky, 1972).

The direct descending influences upon interneurones
are also manifested by facilitation of subthreshold
polysynaptic segmental effects in motoneurones. A vestibulo-spinal volley not strong enough to produce postsynaptic changes in motoneurones, can still facilitate
the appearance of disynaptic IPSP from group Ia afferents in flexor motoneurones (Grillner, Hongo and Lund,

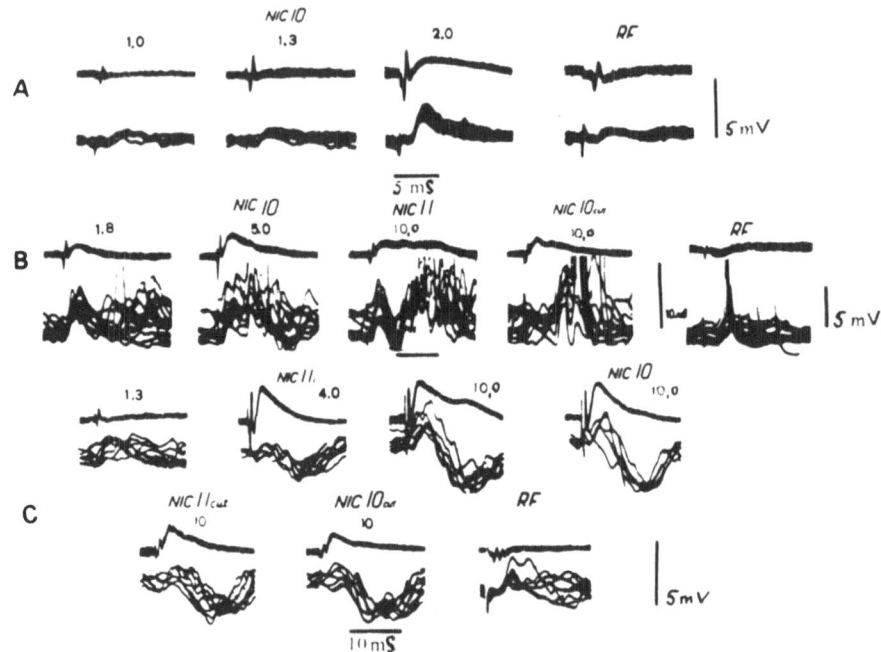

<u>Fig. 11</u>   EPSP and action potentials of 3 segmental
          interneurones (A,B,C) from the medial part of
          the ventral horn, during stimulation of the
          medial part of the medullar reticular forma-
          tion (RF). Effects evoked from different
          branches of the intercostal nerves are also
          presented (Nic), the stimulus strength being
          indicated as multiples of threshold (Bezhenaru,
          Gokin, Zadorozhny and Preobrazhensky, 1972).

1966). Such a volley can also facilitate the transmission of the contralateral extensor reflex (Bruggencate,
Burke, Lundberg and Udo, 1969).

     All these data convey the impression that the
activity of interneurones evoked by the medial descending systems is aimed at strengthening and at expanding
the action already produced directly in motoneurones -
an increase in the extensors' tonus combined with its
decrease in flexor muscles during vestibular signals,
and an increase in flexors' tonus during the reticular
ones.

     More complicated and still in some respect unclear
is the action in spinal cord of volleys coming through
the lateral reticulo-spinal (sometimes called the

"ventral"reticulo-spinal) and the medial vestibulo-
spinal tracts. It is well known, that in the classical
experiments of Magoun and co-workers a concept was established about the existence in the ventro-medial
medullary reticular formation of an unspecific inhibitory system which inhibits all kinds of spinal motor
activity. From the above mentioned data it is obvious
that this inhibition cannot be realized through the

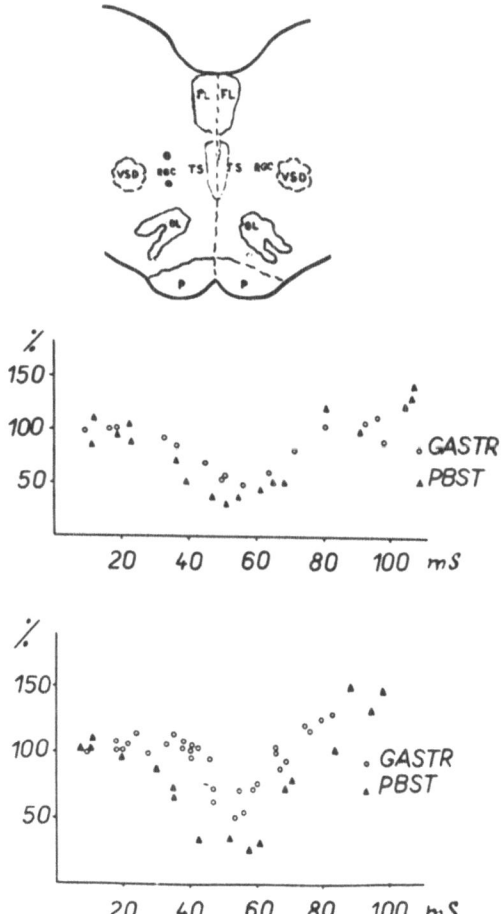

Fig. 12   Changes in the amplitude of ventral root mono-
           synaptic reflex discharges produced by stimula-
           tion of n.gastrocnemius and n.posterior biceps
           + semitendinosus at different intervals after
           stimulation of two points in the central part
           of n.gigantocellularis (location of the stimul-
           ated points is shown at the top) (Kostyuk and
           Preobrazhensky, 1966).

fast-conducting pathways in the medial reticulo-spinal
tract; it has to utilize some other descending structures.
Some data about their origin have been obtained in experiments with local stimulation of different points in
the reticular formation and measurements of changes in
motoneuronal reflex excitability (Kostyuk and Preobrazhensky, 1966). Stimulation of the central and lateral
parts of nucleus gigantocellularis produced very similar
functional changes in all motoneuronal groups (see Fig.
12). The excitability became strongly depressed; the
depression began with a considerable latency (17-20
msec), reached its maximum in 50-55 msec after the onset and lasted about 100 msec (after a short series of
stimuli). Differences in inhibition of flexor and extensor motoneurones were of quantitative nature only,
the inhibition of flexors was, as a rule, more prominent
and long-lasting than that of extensors. The inhibition
could be elicited from both the ipsi- and contralateral
sides. A transsection of the ventro-medial parts of the
lateral funiculus eliminated this effect (sparing the
short-latency responses).

     All mentioned properties of structures that produce
the unspecific inhibition fit well with the characteristics of the lateral reticulo-spinal tract. The nature of
changes in reflex excitability during this inhibition
are complex. On one side long-lasting hyperpolarizing
changes develop both in flexor and extensor motoneurones
(Llinas and Terzuolo, 1964, 1965; Kostyuk and Preobrazhensky, 1966; Jankowska, Lund, Lundberg and Pompeiano,
1968). According to Llinas and Terzuolo, this hyperpolarization shows some differences in flexor and extensor motoneurones. After intracellular chloride injection it shifts to depolarization in extensor motoneurones but not in flexor. However, later investigators
did not confirm this finding.

     On the other side, an additional inhibition of poly-
synaptic transmission to motoneurones also takes place,
based on changes at an interneuronal level. It appears
even in the absence of any hyperpolarizing changes in
motoneurones and has a very long duration as it can be
seen on Fig. 13 (Engberg, Lundberg and Ryall, 1968;
Kostyuk and Preobrazhensky, 1966). The inhibition acts
particularly upon synaptic transmission from the flexor
reflex afferents, but not upon transmission through
interneurones related to group I afferents. A peculiar
property of this inhibition (according to Engberg et al.)
is its disappearance after a transsection of the dorsal
(not ventral) part of the lateral funiculus which does

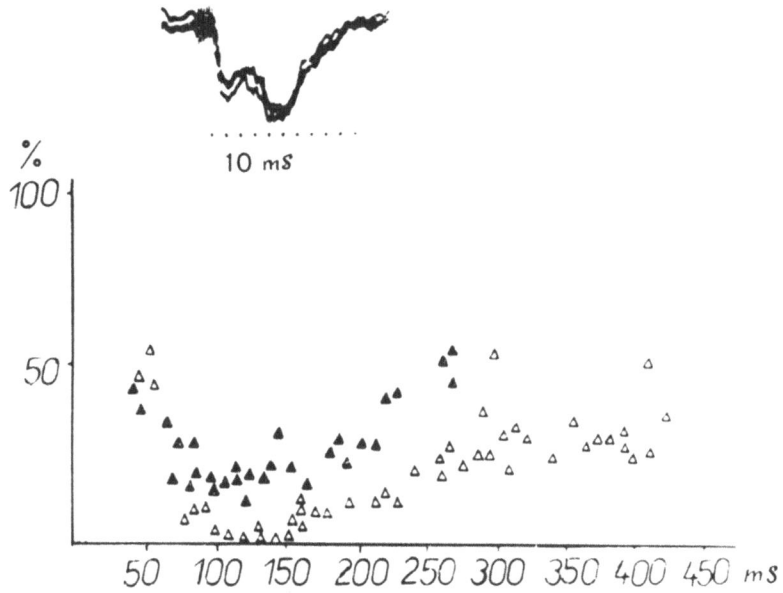

Fig. 13   Variations in the duration of IPSP in an ex-
          tensor motoneurone (A) and of inhibition of
          polysynaptic EPSP (B) in an extensor (black
          triangles) and flexor (white triangles) moto-
          neurone, produced by stimulation of the same
          point of the n.gigantocellularis   (Kostyuk and
          Preobrazhensky, 1967).

not contain morphologically verified reticulo-spinal
pathways. Therefore it was suggested that this action
of the reticular formation is transmitted not through
direct reticulo-spinal fibers but across chains of propriospinal neurones. Even if this suggestion is correct,
the chains cannot be formed by the already mentioned
propriospinal neurones, synaptically connected to the
lateral descending systems. It is important to stress
that usually no descending IPSP could be detected in
interneurones activated by flexor reflex afferents.
Such IPSP's could be found only in a small number of
cells monosynaptically connected to primary afferents.
Perhaps precisely these cells determine the transmission
of afferent volleys to subsequent interneurones.

     The described complex unspecific inhibitory action
of the reticulo-spinal system resembles to a certain
extent the facilitatory action of the lateral systems
on the segmental interneuronal structures and can be
probably considered as some kind of an antagonist of
the latter (although its synaptic mechanisms differ

considerably from the synaptic mechanisms of the lateral systems).

Of course, it is difficult to understand in more
detail the functional meaning of this inhibition in conditions of artificial stimulation. May be, it is more
specific during natural activity and produces certain
reconversions in the functional organization of the
spinal interneuronal apparatus. The changes in the interneuronal activity produced by DOPA can be an example of
the possibility of such reconversion. In spinal cats the
application of this drug produces, like the stimulation
of the lateral reticulo-spinal tract, a depression of
all usual postsynaptic effects evoked by volleys from
high-threshold muscle and cutaneous afferents. Synaptic
effects generated by proprioceptive group I afferents
remain unchanged. At the same time, after DOPA the volleys from flexor afferents begin to elicit quite different effects which are absent in spinal or anesthetiz-
ed animals. A long-lasting excitation of flexor motoneurones appears with great latency on the ipsilateral
side; a parallel excitation of the extensors develops
contralaterally, accompanied by inhibition of the polysynaptic excitation of flexors. Obviously, possibilities
are created for rhythmic alternation of flexor and extensor limb movements: the main component of stepping
(Anden, Jukes, Lundberg and Vyklicky, 1966; Jankowska,
Jukes, Lund and Lundberg, 1967). These authors have suggested that the interneurones which transmit short-
latency effects from flexor reflex afferents tonically
inhibit special interneurones of "long-lasting" action.
This hypothesis has as yet had no direct confirmation.

As far as, according to existing data, DOPA in-
duces an increase of noradrenaline liberation from the
transsected monoamine-ergic descending pathways, a conclusion was made that activity in such pathways is the
factor producing functional reconversions in the spinal
interneuronal system during natural motor activity.
With electric stimulation a selective activation of this
pathway is impossible and the observed results seem to
be quite unspecific.

The function of the medial vestibulo-spinal tract
is still obscure. One part of its fibers exerts an excitatory action upon motoneurones in the cervical segments of the spinal cord. At the same time it contains
fibers producing direct inhibition of motoneurones in
the same segments. Up to now it is the only known example
of inhibitory fibers in the descending pathways, all

other cases of descending inhibition seem to be produced, as already mentioned, by spinal inhibitory interneurones.

     In the beginning we indicated that during natural
motor activity all the descending systems are closely
integrated. They participate in different combinations
in all main forms of motor activity: in defensive and
postural responses, in locomotion and voluntary (conditioned) movements. The most complicated form of motor
activity is presented by voluntary movements. They are
a good example of close functional interconnections
between the descending systems.

     In several investigations it has been shown that
a bilateral section of the pyramidal tract does not produce an irreversible loss of voluntary movements. After
an initial period of disturbances they were almost completely restored. Only the fine movements of the digits
in primates are partially lost. These data indicate
that only the fast-conducting pyramidal fibers which
establish direct contacts with motoneurones of distal
limb muscles in primates are not duplicated by other
pathways. The rest of the cortico-spinal system exerts
its action in association with other parallel systems.
One of them is the cortico-rubro-spinal system, a certain role can be played also by cortico-reticulo-spinal
connections which are established through the medial
reticulo-spinal tract. The possibility that the cortical
motor signal can be transmitted across three different
descending systems does not mean that they are functionally identical. Specific features in the action of each
system can be determined by the different functional
properties of the neurones forming the descending pathways, by the convergence of influences from different
suprasegmental structures participating in the regulation of motor activity and by some special features of
the synaptic connections with the segmental neuronal apparatus. In fact, individual transsections of different
descending pathways can eliminate different components
of the changes in the spinal neuronal apparatus produced
by a cortical volley (Hongo and Jankowska, 1967).

     Of course, interaction of descending systems takes
place also in other forms of motor activity; its nature
is now successfully studied,for instance, during artif-
icially-evoked locomotion in "mesencephalic" cats (Orlovsky and Pavlova, 1972).

Finally, of considerable importance is also the integrative role of the gamma-loop in the coordination of movements. The gamma-motoneurones receive wide influences from the descending systems which often do not coincide with influences upon homonymous alpha-motoneurones. Certainly, this descending control of the activity of stretch receptors through the gamma-motoneurones must be a substantial factor in the regulation of the synaptic excitability of alpha-motoneurones during movements. However, the exact role of the different descending systems in the control of the gamma-loop still needs further elucidation.

REFERENCES

ANDEN N.-E., JUKES M. G. M., LUNDBERG A. and VYKLICKY L. (1966). The effect of DOPA on the spinal cord. I. Influences on transmission from primary afferents. Acta Physiol.scand., 67: 373-386.

ANDERSEN P., ECCLES J. C. and SEARS T. A. (1964). Cortically evoked depolarization of primary afferent fibers in the spinal cord. J.Neurophysiol., 27: 63-77.

BAYEV K. V. and KOSTYUK P. G. (1972 a). Investigation of the modes of connections of cortico- and rubro-spinal tracts with neuronal elements of the servical spinal cord in the cat. Neurophysiology (Kiev), 4: 158-167.

BAYEV K. V. and KOSTYUK P. G. (1972 b). Convergence of cortico- and rubrospinal influences on interneurones of cat cervical spinal cord. Brain Res.,in press.

BEZHENARU I. S., GOKIN A. P., ZADOROZHNY A. G. and PREOBRAZHENSKY N. N. (1972). Synaptic activation of thoracic interneurones by reticulospinal pathways. Neurophysiology (Kiev), 4: in press.

BRUGGENCATE G. ten, BURKE R., LUNDBERG A. and UDO M. (1969). Interaction between the vestibulo-spinal tract, contralateral flexor reflex afferents and Ia afferents. Brain Res., 14: 529-532.

CARPENTER D., LUNDBERG A. and NORRSELL U. (1963). Primary afferent depolarization evoked from the sensorimotor cortex. Acta physiol.scand., 59: 126-142.

ENGBERG I., LUNDBERG A. and RYALL R. W. (1968). Reticulospinal inhibition of transmission in reflex pathways. J.Physiol.(Lond.), 194: 201-223.

GRILLNER S., HONGO T. and LUND S. (1966). Interaction between the inhibitory pathways from the Deiters nucleus and Ia afferents to flexor motoneurones. Acta physiol.scand., 68: suppl. 277.

GRILLNER S. and LUND S. (1966). A descending pathway
    with monosynaptic action in flexor motoneurones. Ex-
    perientia, 22: 390.
GRILLNER S. and LUND S. (1968). The origin of a descend-
    ing pathway with monosynaptic action on flexor moto-
    neurones. Acta physiol.scand., 74: 274-284.
HONGO T. and JANKOWSKA E. (1967). Effects from the
    sensorymotor cortex on the spinal cord in cats with
    transsected pyramids. Exp.Brain Res., 3: 117-137.
JANKOWSKA E., JUKES M. G. M., LUND S. and LUNDBERG A.
    (1967). The effects of DOPA on the spinal cord. V.
    Reciprocal organization of pathways transmitting ex-
    citatory action to alpha motoneurones of flexors and
    extensors. Acta physiol.scand., 70: 369-388.
JANKOWSKA E., LUND S., LUNDBERG A. and POMPEIANO O.
    (1968). Inhibitory effects evoked through ventral
    reticulo-spinal pathways. Archs.ital.Biol., 106: 124-
    140.
KOSTYUK P. G. and MAISKY V. A. (1972). Propriospinal
    projections in the lumbar spinal cord of the cat.
    Brain Res., 39: 530-535.
KOSTYUK P. G., POGORELAYA N. Ch. and DYACHKOVA L. N.
    (1972). Structural features of cortico-spinal connec-
    tions in the cat. Neurophysiology (Kiev), in press.
KOSTYUK P. G. and PREOBRAZHENSKY N. N. (1966). Dif-
    ferentiation of reciprocal and unspecific descending
    synaptic influences during stimulation of the bulbar
    reticular formation. Fiziologichny zhurnal (Kiev),
    12: 712-720.
KOSTYUK P. G. and SKIBO G. G. (1972 a). Structural
    characteristics of the connections of the medial des-
    cending systems with spinal cord neurons. Neurophysio-
    logy (Kiev), 4, in press.
KOSTYUK P. G. and SKIBO G. G. (1972 b). An electron
    microscopic analysis of rubro-spinal tract termina-
    tions in the spinal cord of the cat. Exp.Brain Res.,
    in press.
KOSTYUK P. G., VASILENKO D. A. and LANG E. (1971).
    Propriospinal pathways in the dorso-lateral funiculus
    and their effects on lumbosacral motoneuronal pools.
    Brain Res., 28: 233-249.
KUYPERS H. G. J. M. (1964). The descending pathways to
    the spinal cord, their anatomy and function. Progress
    in Brain Research, 11: 178-202.
LLINAS R. and TERZUOLO C. A. (1964). Mechanisms of
    supraspinal actions upon spinal cord activities.
    Reticular inhibitory mechanisms in alpha extensor
    motoneurones. J.Neurophysiol., 27: 579-590.

LLINAS R. and TERZUOLO C. A. (1965). Mechanisms of
  supraspinal actions upon spinal cord activities.
  Reticular inhibitory mechanisms upon flexor motoneurones. J.Neurophysiol., 28: 413-422.
LLOYD D. (1941). The spinal mechanism of the pyramidal
  system in cats. J.Neurophysiol., 4: 525-546.
LUND S. and POMPEIANO O. (1965). Descending pathways
  with monosynaptic action on motoneurones. Experientia,
  21: 602-603.
LUNDBERG A., NORRSELL U. and VOORHOEVE P. (1962).
  Pyramidal effects on lumbosacral interneurones activated by somatic afferents. Acta Physiol.scand., 56:
  220-229.
NYBERG-HANSEN R. (1966). Functional organization of descending supraspinal fibre systems to the spinal cord.
  Anatomical observations and physiological correla-
  tions. Ergeb.Anat.Entwickl.-Gesch., 39: 1-48.
NYBERG-HANSEN R. and BRODAL A. (1963). Sites of termination of corticospinal fibers in the cat. J.Comp.Neurol.
  120: 369-391.
NYBERG-HANSEN R, and BRODAL A. (1964). Sites and mode of
  termination of rubro-spinal fibers in cat. An experimental study with silver impregnation method. J.Anatomy,
  98: 235-253.
ORLOVSKY G. N. and PAVLOVA G. A. (1972). Vestibular
  responses of neurones of different descending pathways
  in cats with intact cerebellum and in decerebellated
  ones. Neurophysiology (Kiev), 4: 303-310.
PILYAVSKY A. I. and SKIBO G. G. (1969). Relation of the
  rubro-spinal tract with various neurones of the lumbar
  section of the spinal cord. Bull.Eksp.Biol.Med.(USSR),
  68: 3-6.
PREOBRAZHENSKY N. N., BEZHENARU I. S. and GOKIN A. P.
  (1969). Monosynaptic EPSP in thoracic motoneurones
  under reticulo-spinal effect. Neurophysiology (Kiev),
  1: 243-252.
SHAPOVALOV A. I., GRANTYN A. A. and KURCHAVYI G. G.
  (1967). Shortlatency reticulo-spinal synaptic projections to alphamotoneurones. Bull.Eksp.Biol.Med.
  (USSR), 64: 3-9.
SHAPOVALOV A. I., KURCHAVYI G. G. and STROGONOVA M. P.
  (1966). Synaptic mechanisms of vestibulo-spinal influences on alpha-motoneurones. Sechenov Physiol.J.
  USSR, 52: 1401-1409.
VASILENKO D. A. and KOSTYUK P. G. (1965). Activation of
  various groups of spinal neurones in response to
  stimulation of the sensory-motor cortical area in cats.
  Zh.Vysh.Nerv.Deiat.(Moskva), 15: 695-704.

VASILENKO D. A., KOSTYUKOV A. I. and PILYAVSKY A. I.
   (1972). Cortico- and rubrofugal activation of propriospinal interneurones sending axons into the dorso-
   lateral funiculus of the cat spinal cord. Neurophysiology (Kiev), 4: 489-500.
VASILENKO, D. A., ZADOROZHNY A. G. and KOSTYUK P. G.
   (1967). Synaptic processes in the spinal neurones,
   monosynaptically activated by the pyramidal tract.
   Bull.Eksp.Biol.Med. (USSR), 64: 20-25.
WILSON V. J. and YOSHIDA M. (1969 a). Comparison of effects of stimulation of Deiters' nucleus and medial
   longitudinal fasciculus on neck, forelimb and hind-
   limb motoneurones. J.Neurophysiol., 32: 743-758.
WILSON, V. J. and YOSHIDA M. (1969 b). Monosynaptic
   inhibition of neck motoneurones by the medial vestibular nucleus. Exp.Brain Res., 9: 365-380.
ZADOROZHNY A. G., VASILENKO D. A. and KOSTYUK P. G.
   (1970). Pyramidal influences on interneurones of
   spinal reflex arcs in cat. Neurophysiology (Kiev), 2:
   17-25.

CONTROL OF MOTOR ACTIVITY AT THE THALAMIC LEVEL OF THE CAT

ÁNGYÁN, L., L.LÉNÁRD and K.LISSÁK

From the Institute of physiology, Univ.Med.Sch.

Pécs, Hungary

A number of studies have convincingly shown that certain thalamic nuclei are somehow involved in the neural organization of motor behavior.The experimental analysis of complex motor mechanisms at the thalamic level seems to be important considering that co-ordinated complex locomotor patterns - resembling the normal motor activities of the animal - can be elicited by electrical stimulation only at the mesodiencephalic level (Waller, 1940; Hunter and Jasper, 1949; Hess, 1957; Doty, 1961; Koella, 1962; Delgado, 1964; Grastyán, Czopf, Ángyán and Szabó, 1965). In a series of previous experiments using electrical stimulation and different behavioral techniques, characteristic differences were found in the functioning of the anterior and posterior groups of nonspecific thalamic nuclei (Ángyán and Grastyán, 1965; Grastyán and Ángyán, 1967). The aim of the present study was to obtain further information about the role of thalamic nuclei especially in the initiation and performance of a complex locomotor task.

The experiments were carried out on five adult cats. The effects of electrical stimulation and the electrolytic destruction of the same thalamic points were studied with the help of a previously established approach conditioned response. The animals were trained to press a lever to switch on the conditioned sound stimulus (Fig. 1). The lever was placed in the middle of the 180 cm long by 60 cm wide experimental cage. The same kind of feeding devices and loudspeakers were built in the two sides of the cage. The same conditioned sound

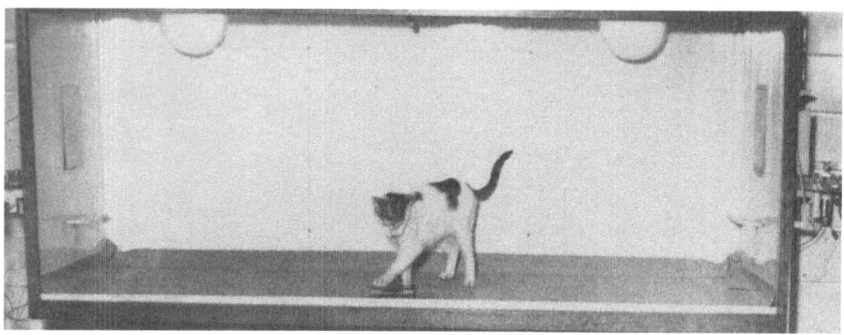

Fig. 1 The cat pressing the lever in the middle of the
        cage to switch on the conditioned sound stimulus

stimulus was variably presented either on the right or
on the left side, thus after pressing the lever in the
middle of the cage the animal had to choose the proper
feeding device to perform a correct response (Fig. 2).
Fifteen trials were given daily to a criterion of 12
correct responses on 4 successive days. After this
criterion was reached, bipolar stainless steel electrodes
were implanted in the anterior, medial and posterior
thalamic regions. The effects of high (100 imp/sec)
frequency stimulation were studied one week after this
operation. There after bilateral electrolytic lesions
were induced by means of the same electrodes: first in
the anterior, one week later in the medial, finally in
the posterior regions.

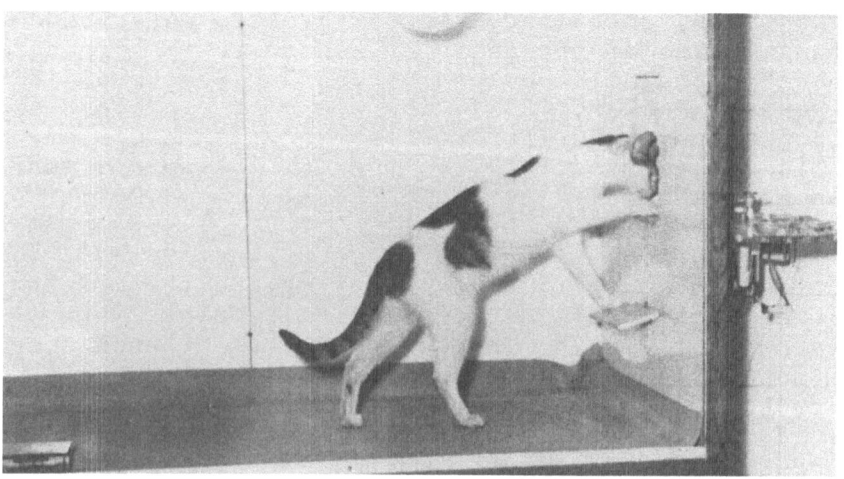

Fig. 2 The cat performing a correct response could take
        out a piece of meat from the feeding device

In agreement with our previous observations
characteristic differences were found between the effects of anterior and posterior thalamic stimulation.
Depending on the stimulation parameters orientation,
tonic motionlessness or contraversive circling often
accompanied by disturbing movements (elevation of the
contralateral forepaw, tilting of the body) were elicited by electrical stimulation of the anterior region
(n.VL-VA). When the conditioned sound stimulus was presented simultaneously with the electrical stimulation
the animal turned immediately to the feeding device and
tried to approach it, but the performance of the conditioned response was deteriorated. A small electrolytic lesion of the same point (Fig. 3A) resulted in an
exaggerated motor activity, but no major disturbance
of the normal behaviour was found. At the presentation
of the conditioned stimulus the animal turned rapidly to
the feeding device and performed the conditioned response with a significantly (p < 0.05) shorter latency
than prior to the induction of the lesion (Fig.4). It
is interesting that even the occurrence of the incorrect
responses decreased (by about 50%) in all animals but
one which on 60 trials made 4 errors prior to and 15
errors after the induction of the lesion.

Stimulation of the region of the dorsomedial
nucleus elicited contraversive circling movements interrupted with motionless periods. The stimulation exerted a suppressing effect on the performance of the conditioned response. Lesions of the dorsomedial nucleus
(Fig.3B), after the previous lesion of the VL-VA area,
produced no conspicuous alterations of the former behavior, except a slight slowing of the performance of
the conditioned response. However, the latencies remained still shorter than in the normal controls (Fig.4).

Stimulation of the posterior region (n.CM) produced
backward and forward locomotion or running. If the animal caught sight of a feeding device during electrical
stimulation, it immediately approached it in absence of
the conditioned stimulus. The simultaneous presentation
of electrical brain and conditional sound stimuli produced and exceedingly short latency response.Small lesions of this point caused minor and inconsistent changes in the latency of the conditioned response.The initiation and the performance of the conditioned response
were significantly suppressed or destroyed only after
a relatively large lesion was induced (Fig.3C).Also the
overt behaviour of the animal changed: longlasting

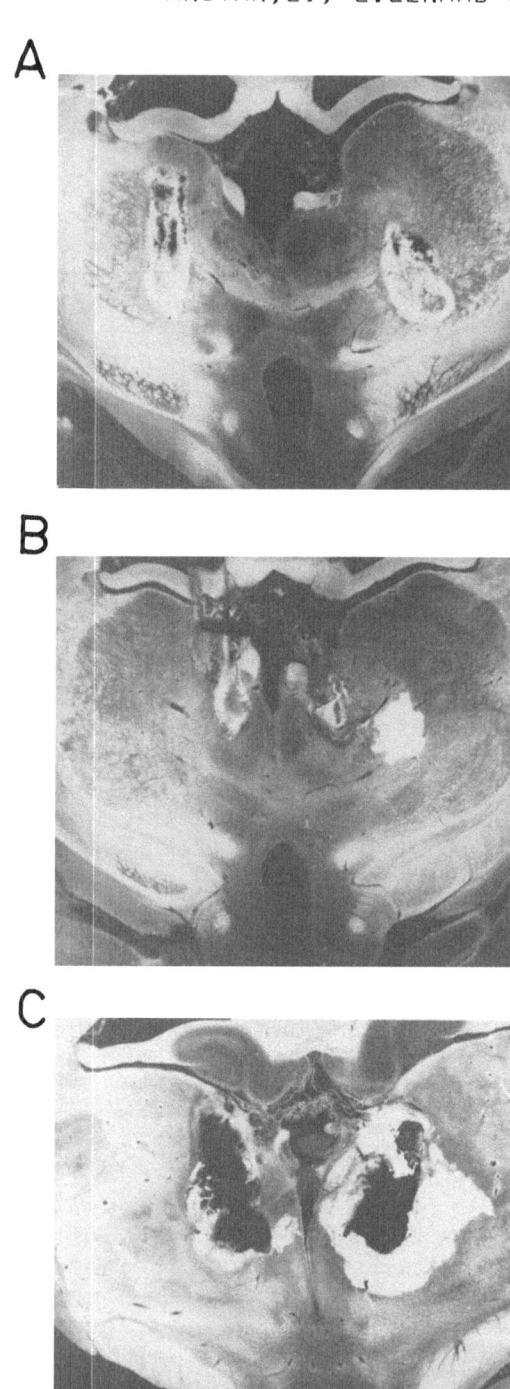

Fig. 3 Brain sections of Cat 2/16 showing locations of the electrolytic lesions in the anterior (A), medial (B) and posterior (C) thalamic regions.

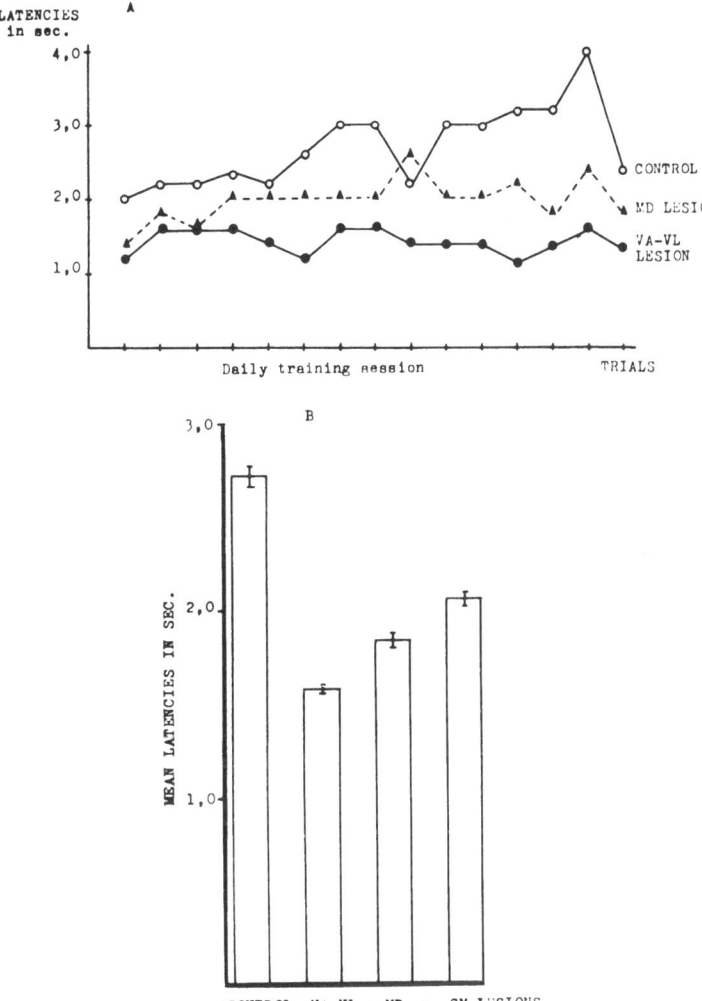

Fig. 4   The effects of thalamic lesions on the latency
          of conditioned response are shown by the curves:
          (A) constructed from latencies measured during
          three typical training sessions, and by the
          columns (B) representing each of them the mean
          latency of 60 responses. (Cat 2/16).

spontaneous locomotion interrupted with motionless periods .- mainly in the corners - was observed. The animal
sometimes knocked against the wall of the cage and could
not recognize the feeding device. However, it could
notice and eat up the meat from a dish placed into the
cage. A slow improvement in the overt behaviour and a
gradual reappearance of the conditioned response was
observed in a few days. However, the latency of the
conditioned response remained much longer than that of
the normal control.

The findings that complex motor patterns may be
elicited by electrical stimulation of thalamic nuclei,
and that the thalamically induced motor activity may be
modulated by an external conditioned stimulus, indicate
that these thalamic structures are closely connected
with both the sensory and the motor system. There are
some data showing that sensory impulses can be conveyed to the motor cortex through anterior thalamic structures (Buser, 1966). In our experiments, the electrical
stimulation of the VA-VL region caused disturbances in
the performance. On the other hand, a relatively small
lesion of the same point produced a significant decrease
of latency of the conditioned response. Both observed
effects might be explained by admitting an inhibitory
mechanism localized in the VA-VL region. The physiological significance of this inhibitory mechanism requires
further studies.

The most remarkable effects were found after the
induction of large bilateral lesions of the posterior
thalamic area. Considering also the powerful facilitating effect of electrical stimulation of the thalamic
centrum medianum it may be supposed that this region represents a natural input of the system. However, the
fact that even after a series of thalamic lesions the
animals are able to perform a previously learned conditioned response let us to conclude that the medial -
thalamic nuclei are not the essential or primary ini-
tiators of complex locomotor activity.

REFERENCES

ÁNGYÁN, L. and E.GRASTYÁN (1965). Some electrical correlates of drive processes elicited from medial thalam-
   ic structures. Acta Physiol.hung. 26: 149-155.
BUSER, P. (1966). Subcortical controls of pyramidal
   activity. In: The Thalamus, ed. D.P.Purpura and M.D.
   Jahr, pp. 323-347. New York: Columbia Univ.Press.
DELGADO, J.M.R. (1964). Free behavior and brain stimula-
   tion. Int.Rev.Neurobiol. 6: 349-449.
DOTY, R.W. (1966). The role of subcortical structures
   in conditioned reflexes. Pavlovian Conference on
   Higher Nervous Activity. Ann.N.Y.Acad.Sci. 92:939-945.
GRASTYÁN, E., J. CZOPF, L. ÁNGYÁN and I.SZABÓ (1965).
   The significance of subcortical motivational mechanisms
   in the organization of conditional connections. Acta
   Physiol.hung. 26: 9-46.

GRASTYÁN, E. and L.ÁNGYÁN (1967). The organization of
   motivation at the thalamic level of the cat. Physiol.
   Behav. 2: 5-13.
HESS, W.R. (1957). The functional organization of the
   diencephalon. New York, Grune and Stratton.
HUNTER, J. and H.H.JASPER(1949). Effects of thalamic
   stimulation in unanaesthetized animals. Electroen.
   Neurophysiol. 1 :305-324.
KOELLA, W.P.(1962). Organizational aspects of some sub-
   cortical motor areas. Int.Rev.Neurobiol. 4: 71-116.
WALLER, W.H. (1940). Progression movements elicited by
   subthalamic stimulation. J.Neurophysiol. 3: 300-307.

MOTOR EFFECTS OF STIMULATION OF THE CEREBRAL CORTEX IN THE DOG. AN ONTOGENETIC STUDY

T. Górska and J.Czarkowska

From the Department of Neurophysiology
Nencki Institute of Experimental Biology
Warsaw, Poland

INTRODUCTION

Electrical stimulation has been applied in studies of the ontogenetic development of the motor cortex by several authors. The results of these experiments are, however, largely controversial. Moreover, the studios have usually focused on the first few weeks of the animal's life, and, therefore, they do not give a full and systematic description of changes taking place in the motor cortex over a longer period of time.

According to some authors (Soltman, 1876; Ferrier, 1880; Tarchanoff, 1878) stimulation of the motor cortex in the dog does not produce movements of skeletal muscles up to the 10th day of life; while, according to others (Paneth, 1885; Michajłow, 1910) the motor cortex is already electrically excitable at birth. Similar results were obtained by Weed and Langworthy (1926) and Henry and Woolsey (1943) in newborn cats.

Different results have also been obtained regarding the sequence of movement appearence in particular parts of the body during the early postnatal period. Paneth (1885) and Soltman (1876) in dogs,and Weed and Langworthy (1926) in cats have found that forelimb movements appear earlier in life than movements of the hindlimb and the face. On the other hand, Henry and Woolsey (1943) in cats have found no time lag between the appearance of facial-masticatory, foreleg and hindleg movements,

all of these responses being present at birth. These
last authors also suggest that the lack of hindleg and
face movements observed in other experiments may have
been due to the fact that appriopriate "centers" of representation of these parts of the body had not been
stimulated.

In view of these controversial results the aim of
the present study was to reinvestigate the problem of
ontogenetic development of the motor cortex in the dog.
Recently Woolsey, Górska, Wetzel, Erickson, Earls and
Allman (1970, 1972), using the electrical stimulation
technique, have analysed in detail the organisation of
the cortical motor areas in the adult dog. Their results,
therefore, made it possible to compare the functions of
the same cortical areas in the adult and young specimen
at various stages of ontogenetic development. Puppies
ranging from 1 day up to 3 months of age were used. It
will be shown that, although movements of particular
parts of the body could be obtained in puppies beginning from their 1st day of life, the process of maturation of the cortical motor areas does not seem to be
completed at the age of 3 months.

In this paper we will confine ourselves to the
analysis of movements produced by stimulation of the
cortical surface of the gyrus sigmoideus posterior and
anterior. Preliminary results have been already published (Górska, Czarkowska and Sybirska, 1972).

MATERIAL AND METHODS

Eighteen puppies from 1 day to 12 weeks of age were
used for the experiments. They were divided into the
following age groups: 1st, 2nd, 3rd, 4th, 6th, 8th,
10th and 12th weeks. In each of these groups experiments
were carried out on 2-3 puppies.

Nembutal (Pentobarbital Sodium) anaesthesia ad-
ministered intraperitoneally was used throughout. The
initial doses ranged from 20 to 40 mg/kg body weight,
depending on the animal's age. Additional doses of 3 mg/
kg were given during the experiment to eliminate spontaneous movements. Atropine 0.1 mg/kg and Fenactil 0.1 mg/kg
premedication was given half an hour before the initial
dose of Nembutal. The rectal temperature was kept at the
optimal level for a given age. Cardiac function was
monitored throughout the experiment. A glass cannula was

inserted into the trachea to allow artificial respiration
when necessary. Details concerning the treatment of
puppies will be described elsewhere (Czarkowska, in
preparation).

The surgical and stimulation methods used in puppies were similar to those for adult dogs (Woolsey et
al., 1970, 1972). The dorsolateral surface of the cortex
over the sigmoid gyri was exposed. Warm physiological
saline was used to prevent drying of the pial surface.
The animals body was supported horizontally with limbs
pendant in order to allow maximal freedom of movement.
The head was fixed rigidly in a special headholder.

Unipolar stimulation with a stainless steel electrode of 0.5 mm in diameter was used throughout. The indifferent electrode was attached to a saline soaked ring
placed on the animal's scalp. A 50 cps sine wave current
was delivered through a high impedance device, the intensity of the current was monitored by a milliampere
meter. The duration of each stimulation was 2.5 sec,and
the minimal interval between successive stimulations was
2 min (Woolsey, Settlage, Meyer, Sencer, Pinto-Hamuy and
Travis, 1952).

The exposed cortex was explored in 2 mm steps. The
position of each point was marked on an enlarged photo-
graph of the brain. Each point was stimulated several
(at least 3) times in order to determine the threshold
value of stimulation producing visible movement and to
analyze movements recruited with suprathreshold stimulation (up to 150% of the threshold value). The maximal
value of stimulation used in puppies was 5.0 mA.

At least three investigators participated in observation of movements elicited by cortical stimulation.
The results of each stimulation were analyzed and described in detail. Special attention was paid to proper
estimation of the strength, sequence and character of
movements.

At the termination of the experiment the animal was
given an extradose of Membutal and perfused with 0.9%
saline followed by 10% formol. The brain was then re-
moved from the skull and photographed in standard views.

The method of figurine maps elaborated by Woolsey
and his co-workers (Woolsey et al., 1952; Welker, Benjamin, Miler and Woolsey, 1957; Hardin, Arumugasamy and

Jameson, 1968) has been used for illustration of the results. On each figurine the muscle group or body part engaged in the movement is marked. The symbols of various kinds of movements are similar to those used by Welker et al. (1957). Each figurine corresponds to one cortical point stimulated. Unilateral figurines represent the contralateral side of the animal. In order to maintain the appropriate direction of individual figurines within the pattern of somatotopic organization of sensory (SI) and motor areas, right-sided figurines were used for area SI (Pinto-Hamuy, Bromley and Woolsey, 1956) and left-sided figurines for the motor cortex. In bilateral figurines the contralateral side of the body is marked on the corresponding part of the figurine according to the convention used for unilateral figurines, and the mirror-image half of the figurines represents the ipsilateral side of the animal.

A variety of symbols has been used for denoting various features of movements obtained in puppies. In adult-like forms of responses solid black represents the earliest, strongest or lowest-threshold movement; hatched, intermediate grades; and small dots, the weakest or highest-threshold movement elicited. These symbols also indicate that movements were tonic and repetitive, that is successive stimulations of the same cortical point yielded similar motor responses.

For other movements specific for puppies, the following symbols are used. An interrupted line denotes a variable response which could not be repeated on successive stimulation of the same cortical point. A solid line indicates a repetitive movement. Repetitive responses elicited at threshold value of stimulation are marked by large dots, and dashed hatching means a repetitive response recruited with suprathreshold stimulation. A solid line without any pattern inside denotes a movement which we could not classify, for some reason, as repetitive or variable.

The following symbols have been used to describe the character of movements in puppies: J - for jerk-like, P - for phasic, C - for clonic, CT - for clonic with a tonic component, T - for a tonic movement. Arrows between letters mean that increasing strength of stimulation caused a change in the character of the response, i.e. from a jerk-like into a phasic or tonic.

RESULTS

Motor effects elicited by cortical stimulation in puppies appeared to be largely different from those of adult animals. These differences are best seen when the results obtained in puppies are compared with the results in adult dogs. Therefore, we shall first give a short review of the characteristics of movements elicited by stimulation of the gyrus sigmoideus posterior and anterior in the adult dog.

1. Motor Effects of Cortical Stimulation
in Adult Dogs

Fig. 1 illustrates movements obtained on stimulation of the gyrus sigmoideus posterior and anterior in adult dogs. Examination of this figure reveals several characteristic features of these responses.

First, stimulation of various parts of the cortex yields movements of different parts of the body, which shows that the motor cortex of the dog is somatotopically organized. As illustrated in Fig. 1, stimulation of medial parts of the gyrus sigmoideus posterior produced movements of the hindlimbs (see hind-quarter figurines), and stimulation of lateral parts of this gyrus and of gyrus sigmoideus anterior elicited forelimb movements (forequarter figurines). In between there was a zone from which both fore- and hindlimbs movements were evoked.

Among movements of the hindlimbs, knee flexion, thigh protraction and ankle dorsiflexion were most frequently observed, and these movements were elicited from relatively large cortical regions. Other movements, such as thigh retraction, knee extension, flexion and extension of toes occurred less frequently and were elicited from more limited cortical areas. As for foreleg movements, elbow flexion, arm retraction and wrist dorsiflexion predominated. Finger movements, wrist flexion and elbow extension were seen less frequently. Trunk movements could be elicited from rostral parts of the anterior sigmoid gyrus. From the same area movements of arm protraction were produced as well. Stimulation of the gyrus sigmoideus posterior did not produce trunk movements in adult dogs.

Another typical feature of movements produced by

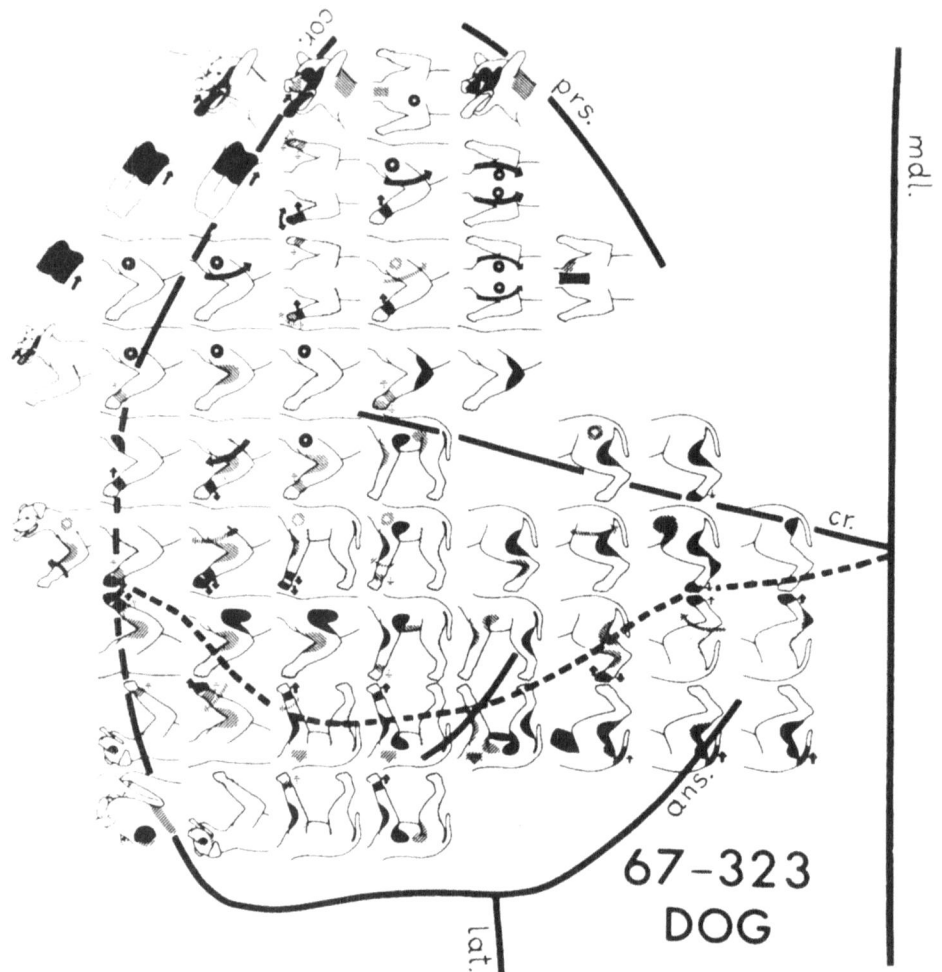

Fig. 1 Figurine map to illustrate the movements elicit-
        ed by electrical stimulation of the gyrus sig-
        moideus posterior and anterior of the left hemi-
        sphere in an adult dog. The heavy solid lines
        indicate sulci. The heavy dashed line indicate
        the boundary between the somatic sensory (SI)
        and the motor area. Prs-presylvian sulcus; Cr-
        cruciate sulcus; ans-ansate sulcus; lat-lateral
        sulcus; cor-coronal sulcus; mdl-midline. For
        explanation of symbols see Methods.

stimulation of the motor cortex in adult dogs is the
predominance of contralateral responses. As shown in
Fig. 1, stimulation of the whole gyrus sigmoideus posterior yielded exclusively movements of the contralateral

parts of the body (see one-sided figurines). These movements were also relatively discrete and simple. i.e. at
threshold stimulation they were limited to one or two
joints only. Stimulation of the gyrus sigmoideus anterior
elicited bilateral movements (bilateral figurines) in
addition to contralateral movements. Responses produced
from this region were also more complex than those obtained from the gyrus sigmoideus posterior, i.e. they
usually involved all joints of the limb.

Movements elicited by cortical stimulation in adult
dogs could be classified as tonic ones. This means that
they appeared with a relatively short latency and lasted
throughout the period of stimulation. Also these responses were generally repetitive, that is successive
stimulation of the same cortical point yielded essentially similar movements. As explained above (see method),
all symbols used in Fig. 1, mean that the motor reactions were both tonic and repetitive.

The lowest-threshold values of stimulation were observed near the lateral end of the cruciate sulcus. In
this area threshold values ranged from 0,2 mA to 0,5 mA.
More medially the values were higher, up to 1,0 mA. In
the remaining areas, that is in the gyrus sigmoideus
anterior and area SI (Pinto-Hamuy et al., 1956) thresholds ranged from 1,0 mA to 3,0 mA.

2. Motor Effects of Cortical Stimulation
in Puppies

Stimulation of the motor cortex in puppies evoked
movements of skeletal muscles beginning from the first
day of life. However, for a long period of time these
movements were significantly different from motor responses obtained in adult dogs. Two periods in the development of the motor cortex in puppies could be differentiated:

A. The period from birth to the fourth week of life,
   when movements in puppies were essentially different
   from those elicited in adult dogs.

B. The period from the 4th week of life to about three
   months, when movements in puppies gradually took on
   the appearance of the movements in adult dogs. Movements elicited during both these periods of life are
   described:

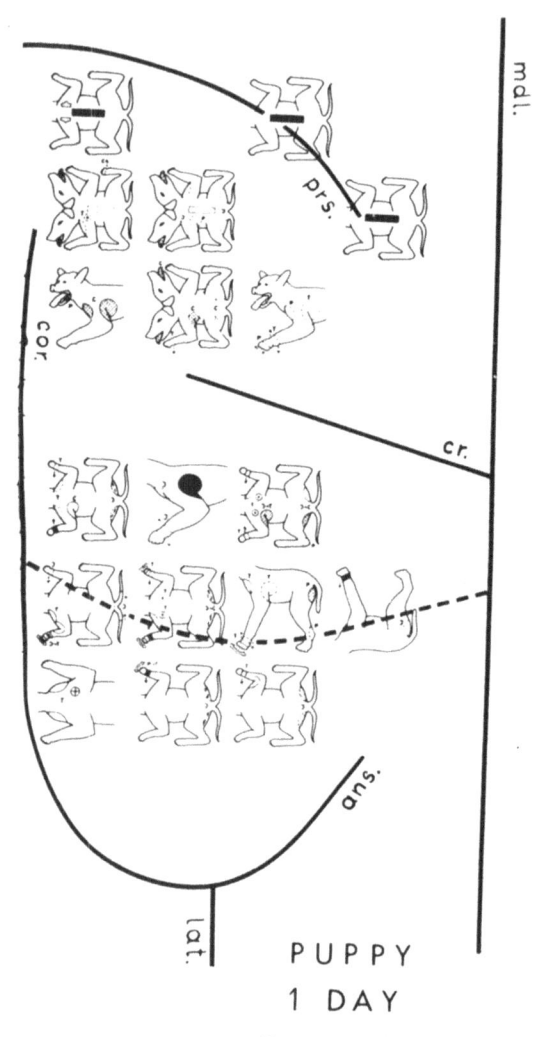

PUPPY
1 DAY

(S.1.M X X I X .12 X I 71)

Fig 2   Figurine map to illustrate the movements elicit-
         ed by electrical stimulation of the gyrus sigmo-
         ideus posterior and anterior of the left hemi-
         sphere in a 1 day-old puppy. Abbreviations as
         in Fig. 1.

    A. The period from birth to the 4th week of life
    Fig. 2 and 3 illustrate movements elicited on
stimulation of the sigmoid gyri in puppies 1 day and
13 days old, respectively. Comparison of these figures
with Fig. 1 indicates several differences in the responses of puppies of this age as compared with adult
dogs.

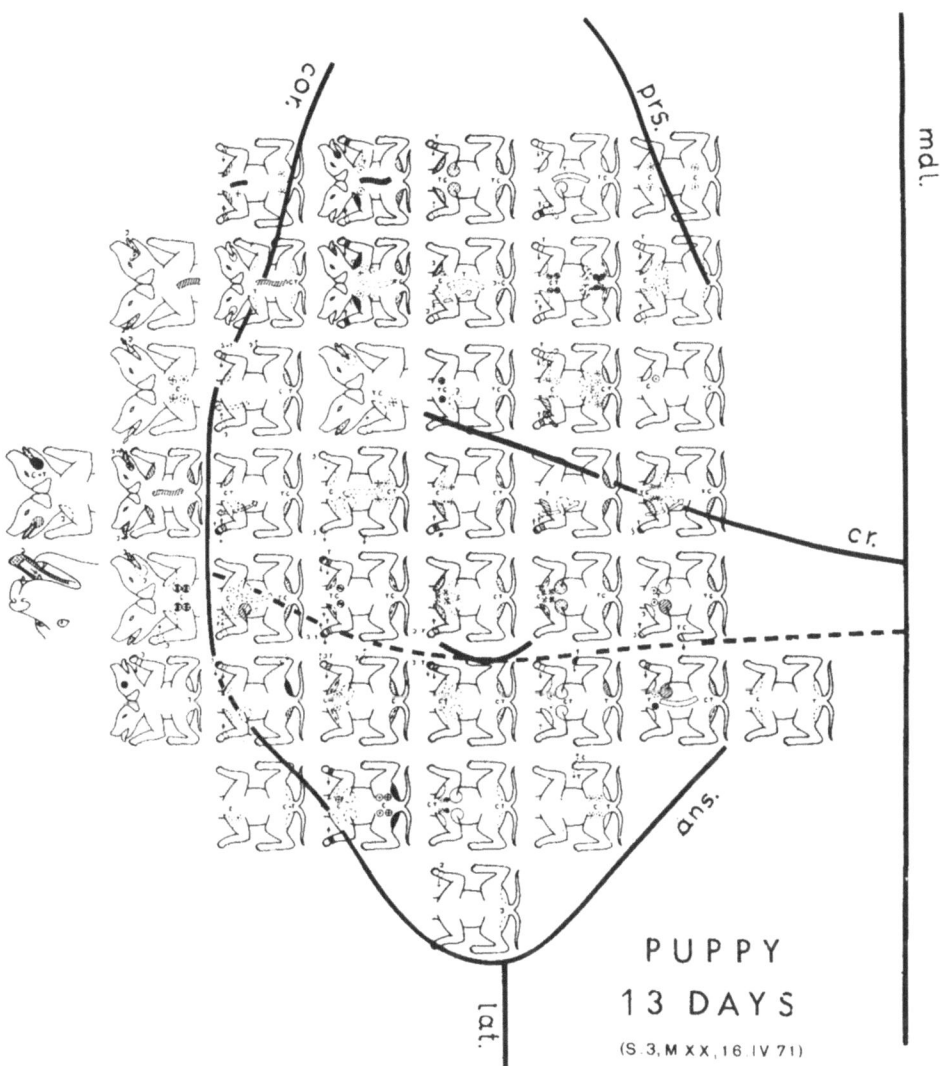

Fig. 3   Figurine map to illustrate the movements elicit-
         ed by electrical stimulation of the gyrus sigmo-
         ideus posterior and anterior of the left hemi-
         sphere in a 13 days old puppy. Abbreviations as
         in Fig. 1.

     The first characteristic feature of this period
was the lack of somatotopic organization of the motor
cortex. Whereas in the adult dog there is a clear somatotopic organization of the motor cortex, with hindlimb
representation lying more medially, and forelimb, more
laterally; in puppies up to the 4th week of life stimula-

tion of any part of the cortex in a mediolateral direction usually elicited movements of both fore- and hindlimbs. This difference is easily seen when comparing
Fig. 1 with Fig. 2 and 3. In Fig. 1 the medial and lateral parts of the map are covered with figurines representing the hind- and forequarters respectively, but in
Fig. 2 and 3 almost the whole area is covered with figurines representing both fore- and hindquarters.

Another feature of the movements in puppies of this
age was the bilaterality of motor responses. In adult
dogs bilateral movements were obtained on stimulation
of the gyrus sigmoideus anterior , but stimulation of
the gyrus sigmoideus posterior yielded contralateral
responses only. In puppies, however, stimulation of the
sigmoid gyri yielded in the majority of cases movements
in both the ipsi- and contralateral sides. This is illustrated in Fig. 2 and 3 by a great number of bilateral
figurines, as compared with unilateral figurines pre-
dominating in Fig. 1.

An additional difference between puppies of this
age and adult animals was the relatively meager repertory of movements observed in puppies. As seen in Fig 2
and 3, in puppies up to the 4th week of age the majority
of movements occurred in the proximal joints. Hindlimb
movements were essentially limited to reaction of the
thigh, which in adult animals occurs relatively rarely.
In the case of the forelimbs, the variety of movements
was greater, including retraction, protraction, abduc-
tion and adduction at the shoulder, as well as wrist
dorsiflexion and extension of fingers. Other movements
typical for adult dogs, such as thigh protraction, knee
and elbow flexion, could not usually be elicited by cortical stimulation in this period of life.

The last difference between the movements elicited
in adult dogs and puppies up to the 4th week of age concerns the character of the movements. In adult dogs
movements elicited by cortical stimulation were virtually always tonic and repetitive (see above). On the contrary, in puppies up to the 4th week of age movements
were, in general, neither tonic nor repetitive. As it
is shown in Fig. 2 and 3, the majority of movements were
either jerk-like, phasic, clonic or clonic with a tonic
component. These categories of movements are indicated
in Fig. 2-6 by appropriate letters (see Methods). Sometimes increasing strengh of stimulation caused a change
in the character of the movement, i.e. from jerk-like
into phasic or tonic (arrows between letters). These

movements were also quite variable, i.e. successive
stimulation of the same cortical point produced different responses from stimulation to stimulation. As seen

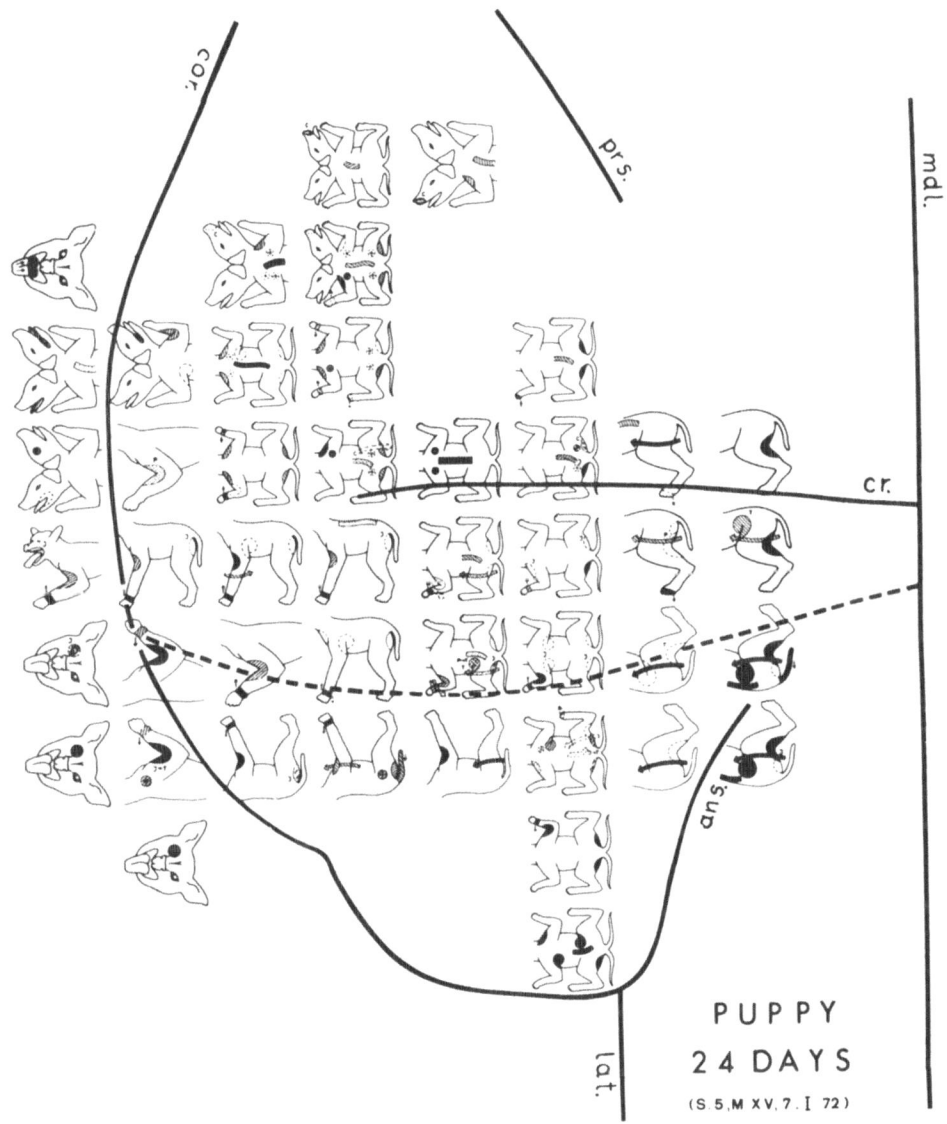

Fig. 4   Figurine map to illustrate the movement elicited
          by electrical stimulation of the gyrus sigmoid-
          eus posterior and anterior of the left hemi-
          sphere in a 24 days old puppy. Abbreviations as
          in Fig. 1.

in Fig. 2 and 3, stimulation of the cortex yielded variable responses at the majority of points (interrupted
line), the number of repetitive responses (solid line)
being relatively small.

B. The period from the 4th to 12th week of life
An essential change in movements evoked by electrical stimulation of the motor cortex took place in puppies
at the transition from the 3rd to the 4th week of their
life. Beginning from the 4th week onward some adult-like
features of movements began to appear and then develop
gradually. This process lasted at least until the 12th
week of life.

Fig. 4, 5 and 6 show the results of mapping the
motor cortex in puppies 24, 40 and 83 days of age, respectively.

As is shown in Fig. 4, in a 24 days old puppy a
somatotopic organization of the motor cortex is beginning to appear. Stimulation of the medial part of the
gyrus sigmoideus posterior produced movements to the
hindquarters only. In the lateral part of the gyrus
sigmoideus posterior foreleg movements began to dominate.
In between there is a zone yielding movements of both
fore- and hindquarters.

In parallel with this shift toward a somatotopic
organization a process of gradual development of contralateral representation of the animal's body was observed. Stimulation of the gyrus sigmoideus posterior began
to evoke movements of the contralateral extremities
mainly (see ipsilateral figurines in Fig. 4, 5 and 6).
Bilateral movements of the extremities were gradually
limited to a zone in the middle part of the gyrus
sigmoideus posterior (Fig. 4 and 5). In a puppy 83 days
old (Fig. 6), bilateral movements had almost completely
disappeared from the gyrus sigmoideus posterior. They
were mainly obtained from the gyrus sigmoideus anterior,
the latteral being the area from which bilateral movements are obtained in the adult dog as well.

At the same time an increase in the diversity of
movements elicited by cortical stimulation was observed.
Movements of knee flexion and thigh protraction began
to appear (Fig. 4) and then to dominate (Fig. 6). Movements of toes and ankle were also observed (see Fig. 6).
In the case of foreleg movements the number of shoulder
protractions began to decrease, and movements of shoulder

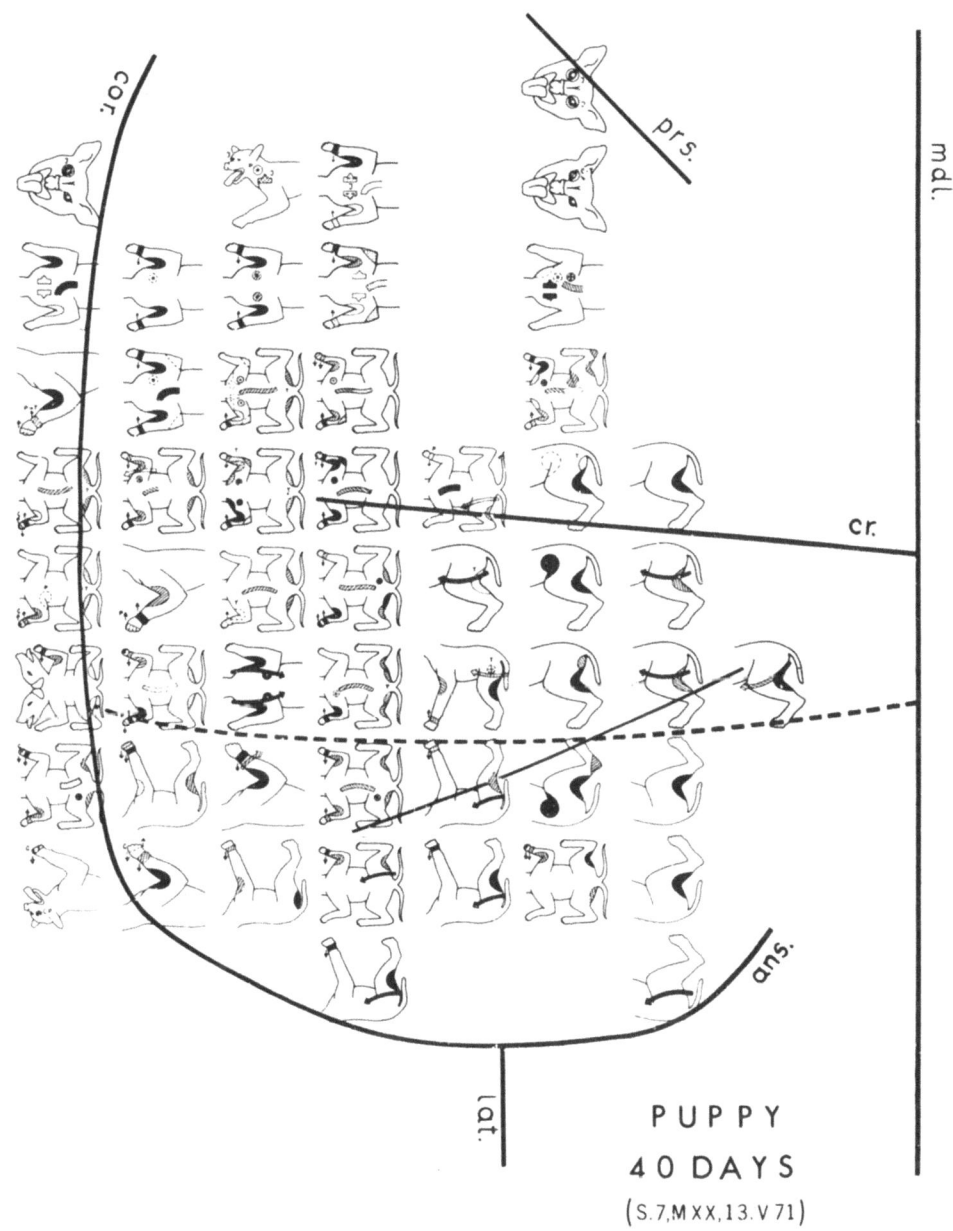

<u>Fig. 5</u>   Figurine map to illustrate the movements elicit-
         ed by electrical stimulation of the gyrus sigmoid-
         eus posterior and anterior of the left hemi-
         sphere in a 40 days old puppy. Abbreviations as
         in Fig. 1.

retraction increased, the picture resembling that of an

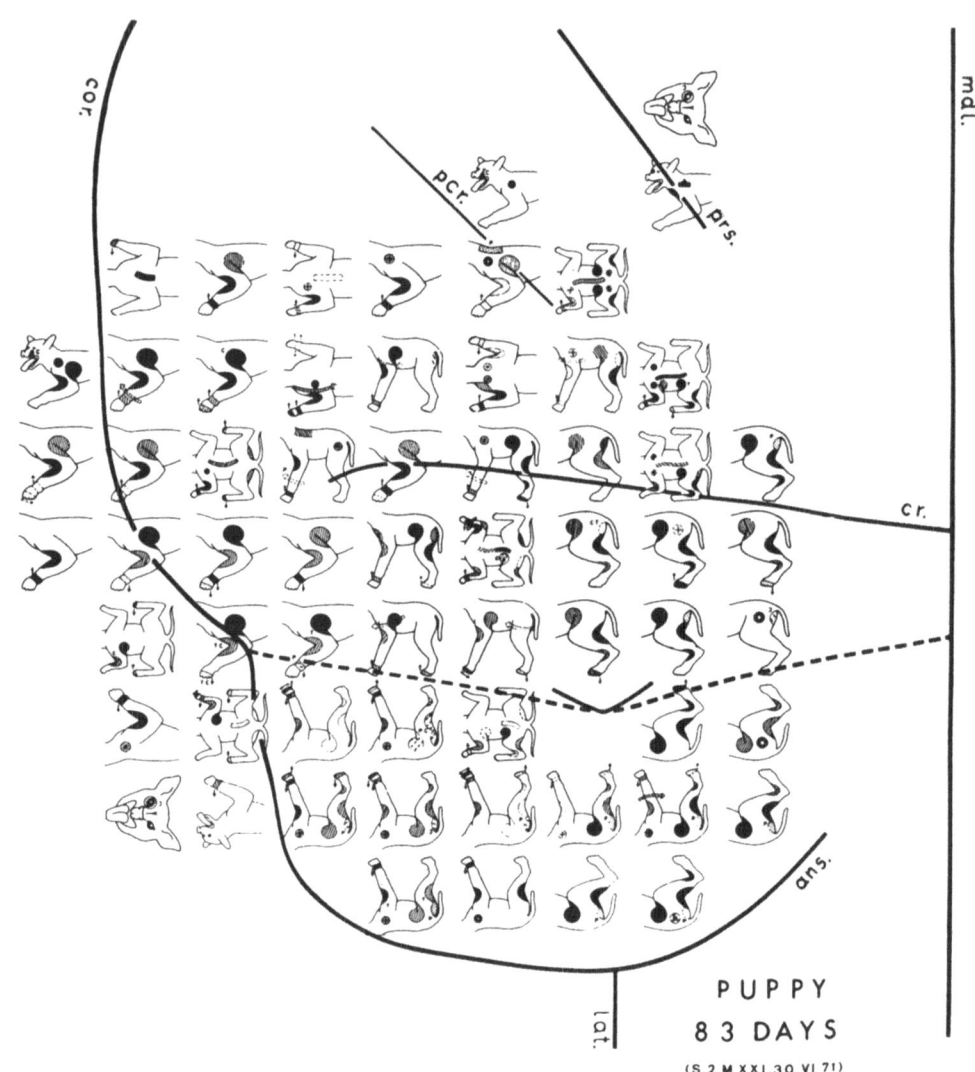

Fig. 6   Figurine map to illustrate the movements elicit-
         ed by electrical stimulation of the gyrus sigmo-
         ideus posterior and anterior in a 83 days old
         puppy. Abbreviations as in Fig. 1.

adult animal.   Movements of elbow flexion, as well as
wrist and finger flexion were also often encountered.

     Special attention should be paid to trunk movements
observed in puppies in this period. In adult dogs trunk
movements appear on stimulation of the anterior sigmoid

gyrus. In puppies, however, these movements were also
fairly often elicited from the middle parts of the gyrus
sigmoideus posterior. The cortical area from which trunk
movements were evoked decreased with age. At the end of
the 3rd month (Fig. 6) trunk movements were limited to
the anterior sigmoid gyrus, as in the adult dog (compare
Fig. 1).

Beginning at the 4th week the character of movements in puppies also began to change. Instead of jerk-
like, phasic, or clonic responses, tonic movements began
to dominate. Moreover, responses began to be repetitive.
In Figs. 4, 5 and 6 the number of symbols denoting movements other than tonic (J, P, C, CT) and variable (interrupted line) gradually decreases, and the number of
symbols denoting tonic and repetitive movements increases, reminding the pattern of the adult dog (compare
Fig. 1).

Although our experiments were not carried out on
puppies older than 12 weeks, our data suggest that the
process of gradual maturation of the movements is not
completed at the end of the 3rd month of life. Comparison of Fig. 6 and 1 shows that in 12 weeks old puppies
the area from which foreleg movements could be obtained
was smaller than in adult animals. This suggests that
the representation of the foreleg may not be fully developed at this period yet. Moreover, the threshold
values of stimulation were higher in puppies than in
adult animals. Whereas in adult dogs the lowest threshold values ranged between 0.2 mA and 0.5 mA, in puppies
12 weeks old thresholds below 0.5 mA were rarely seen.

DISCUSSION

The results described above confirm findings of
previous authors (Paneth, 1885; Michajłow, 1910), showing that in the dog the motor cortex is electrically excitable at birth. They also support the evidence indicat-
ing that, not only fore-limb movements but also hind-
limb movements could be elicited at birth by cortical
stimulation (Henry and Woolsey, 1943).

A comparison of movements produced by electrical
stimulation of the motor cortex in adult dogs and puppies of different age led us to differentiate two periods
in the ontogenetic development of the motor cortex in
the dog: an early one from birth up to approximately

the fourth week of life, and a later one, from the
fourth week of life to at least 3 months. In the first
period movements evoked by cortical stimulation were
quite different from those of adult animals. The main
features of this period are lack of somatotopic organization of the motor cortex, lack of dominant representation of the contralateral parts of the body and a meager
repertory of movements. Moreover, movements elicited in
this period were only rarely tonic and repetitive. These
latter features have been also noticed by other authors
(Paneth, 1885 b); Michajłow, 1910; Kennard and McCulloch,
1942).

Beginning with the fourth week a process of gradual
maturation of movements elicited by cortical stimulation
is observed. Somatotopic organization and contralateral
representation of the body first make their appearance
and then gradually evolve in the direction of the adult
pattern. The repertory of movements is enriched, resembling that of adult animals. Also, movements become tonic
and repetitive on successive stimulation of the same
cortical point. At the end of the third month the general picture of movements produced by electrical stimulation of the motor cortex becomes essentially similar to
that in adult animals. However, some minor differences
are still present, suggesting that the process of maturation of the motor cortex is not yet completed at this
age.

The importance of the fourth week of life of puppies with regard to the development of adult-like patterns of motor reactions has been stressed by several
authors. A normal distribution of muscle tone appears in
this period, which causes the disappearance of tremor
and oscillations during standing and walking (James,
1952; Fox, 1963, 1964). Several reflexes typical for
very young animals decline in the fourth week, and reflexes typical for adult animals appear instead (Fox,
1963, 1964, 1971). Puppies of this age begin to run. The
EEG pattern in puppies in the fourth week begins to resemble closely that of an adult animal (Dipperi, Himwich and Peterson, 1964). All these changes are probably
connected with the process of extensive myelinization of
the nervous system, taking place in this period (Dravid
and Himwich, 1964; Dmitrieva and Kalinina, 1965).

Changes in the pattern of motor responses elicited
by cortical stimulation in puppies beginning with the
fourth week of age may be partly related with the process

of maturation of the corticospinal tract. At the age
of three weeks all tracts in the spinal cord of a dog
are myelinated with the exception of the lateral cortico-
spinal tract and the fasciculus gracilis, in which the
myelinization is completed at the age of six weeks (Fox,
Inman and Himwich, 1967). The postnatal development of
the spinal terminations of the corticospinal tract lasts,
however, much longer, achieving by the age of three
months a pattern of projection similar to but not yet
identical with that found in the adult dog (Buxton and
Goodman, 1967). Similar conclusions regarding the duration of maturation of the corticospinal tract could be
drawn from measurements of conduction velocities of
corticospinal fibers in puppies of different age (Kirk
and Breazile, 1972). They are in agreement with our results showing that in the dog the maturation of the
motor cortex is not yet completed at the end of the
third month.

In macaques the process of maturation of the corticospinal tract is not yet over at the age of eight
months (Kuypers, 1962) and this would correspond to the
results of cortical stimulation experiments, showing
that in infant monkeys the extent of the motor cortex
and the threshold current producing movements approach
the value of the adult animal at the age of one year
and over (Boynton and Hines, 1933). These differences
in time reflect differences in the degree of corticalization of motor functions in the various species. They
are in agreement with the data showing greater functional significance of the pyramidal tract in monkeys (Tower,
1940; Lawrence and Kuypers, 1965; Wiesendanger, 1969;
Górska et al., 1972) as compared with dogs (Górska, 1967;
Joffe and Samoylov, 1971) and cats (Górska, Jankowska
and Mossakowski, 1966 a, b; Laursen and Wiesendanger,
1966; Voneida, 1967; Wiesendanger, 1969).

Further experiments are presently carried out in
order to evaluate the functional significance of the
pyramidal tract at various stages of ontogenetic development of the dog.

The authors are greatly indebted to Mrs. I.Malinow-
ska and Mrs. E.Sybirska for their helpful assistance
in the experiments.

SUMMARY

In puppies ranging from 1 day to 3 months of age
the posterior and anterior sigmoid gyri were stimulated
under Nembutal anaesthesia and the movements obtained
were analyzed. Monopolar stimulation of controlled intensity, 50 cps was used. It was found that movements
of the extremities elicited by cortical stimulation,
although present in newborn animals, did not resemble
at all those of adult dogs. Whereas in adult dogs
stimulation of the motor cortex usually produces relatively simple, tonic movements of the contralateral extremities with a clear somatotopic distinction between fore-
and hindlimb representations, movements obtained in
puppies in their first 3 weeks of life were jerk-like,
clonic or phasic, and involved all four extremities.
Beginning with the 4th week adult-like features of movements appeared in puppies and then developed gradually.
At the end of the 3rd month, movements in puppies were
essentially similar to those of adult dogs. However,
some minor differences were still present, suggesting
that the process of maturation of the motor cortex is not
yet completed at this age.

REFERENCES

BOYNTON E. P. and HINES M. (1933). On the question of
    threshold in stimulation of the motor cortex. Am.J.
    Physiol. 56: 170-174.
BUXTON D. F. and GOODMAN D. C. (1967). Motor function
    and the corticospinal tracts in the dog and raccoon.
    J.Comp.Neurol. 129: 341-360.
DIPERRI R., HIMWICH W. A. and PETERSON J. (1964). The
    evolution of the EEG in the developing brain of the
    dog. In: Progress in Brain Res. 9: 89-92.
DMITRIEVA N. I. and KALININA E. I. (1965). Myeliniza-
    tion of the central auditory path with postnatal onto-
    genesis in the dog. J.Evolution Bioch.Physiol. 1:
    193-198.
DRAVID A. R. and HIMWICH W. A. (1964). Biochemical
    studies of the central nervous system of the dog dur-
    ing maturation. In: Progress in Brain Res. 9: 170-173.
FERRIER D. (1880). The functions of the brain. New York:
    Putnam's.
FOX H. W. (1963). The development and clinical signific-
    ance of muscle tone and posture in the neonate dog.
    Am.J.Vet.Res, 24: 1232-1239.

FOX H. W. (1964). The ontogeny of behaviour and neuro-
    logic responses in the dog. Animal Behaviour, 12: 301-
    311.
FOX H. W. (1971). Integrative development of brain and
    behaviour in the dog. Chicago and London: The Univers-
    ity of Chicago Press.
FOX H. W., INMAN O. R. and HIMWICH W. A. (1967). The
    postnatal development of the spinal cord of the dog.
    J.Comp.Neurol. 130: 233-240.
GÓRSKA T., JANKOWSKA E. and MOSSAKOWSKI M. (1966 a).
    Effects of pyramidotomy on instrumental conditioned
    reflexes in cats. I.Manipulatory reflexes. Acta Biol.
    Exp. (Warsaw), 26: 335-344.
GÓRSKA T., JANKOWSKA E. and MOSSAKOWSKI M. (1966 b).
    Effects of pyramidotomy on instrumental conditioned
    reflexes in cats. II. Reflexes derived from uncondi-
    tioned reactions. Acta Biol.Exper. (Warsaw),26:345-356.
GÓRSKA T. (1967). Instrumental conditioned reflexes
    after pyramidotomy in dogs. Acta Biol.Exper.(Warsaw),
    27: 103-121.
GÓRSKA T., CZARKOWSKA J. and SYBIRSKA E. (1972). Onto-
    genetic development of cortical motor representation
    in dogs. In: Proc.XII Congr.Polish Physiol.Soc.
    (Olsztyn), Abstr.of free commun. 75.
HARDIN W. B., ARUMUGASAMY N. and JAMESON H. D. (1968).
    Pattern of localization in "precentral" motor cortex
    of raccoon. Brain Research, 11: 611-627.
HENRY E.W. and WOOLSEY C. N. (1943). Somatic motor re-
    sponses produced by electrical stimulation of the
    cerebral cortex of new-born and young kittens. Fed.
    Proc.Amer.Soc.Exp.Biol. 2: 21.
JAMES W. T. (1952). Observations on the behaviour of
    new-born puppies: II summary of movements involved
    in group orientation. J.Comp.Psychol.Physiol. 45:
    329-335.
JOFFE M. E. and SAMOYLOV M. J. (1971). On the inter-
    action of the pyramidal and the rubrospinal system
    in the regulation of local movements. In: Mechanism
    of descending control of spinal cord activities.Trans.
    of the 3rd Symposium on General Physiology, Kiev,1968,
    ed. P. G. Kostyuk, 143-144, Leningrad: Nauka.
KENNARD M. A. and McCULLOCH W. S. (1942). Excitability
    of cerebral cortex in infant Macaca Mulatta. J.Neuro-
    physiol. 5: 231-234.
KIRK G. R. and BREAZILE J. E. (1972). Maturation of the
    corticospinal tract in the dog. Expl.Neurol. 35: 394-
    397.
KUYPERS H. G. J. M. (1962). Corticospinal connections:
    Postnatal development in the Rhesus Monkey. Science,
    138: 678-680.

LAURSEN A. M. and WIESENDANGER M. (1966). Motor deficits
    after transection of a bulbar pyramid in the cat.
    Acta physiol.scand. 68: 118-126.
LAWRENCE D. G. and KUYPERS H. G. J. M. (1965). Pyramidal
    and nonpyramidal pathways in monkeys. Anatomical and
    functional correlation. Science, 148: 973-975.
MICHAJŁOW S. (1910). Zur Frage über die Erregbarkeit der
    motorischen Zentra in der Hirnrinde neugeborener Soiuge-
    tiere. Pflüg.Arch.ges.Physiol. 133: 45-70.
PANETH I. (1885). Ueber Lage, Ausdehnung und Bedeutung
    der absoluten motorischen Felder auf der Hirnoberfläche
    des Hundes. Arch.f.d.ges.Physiol., 37: 523-561.
PINTO-HAMUY T., BROMILEY H. B. and WOOLSEY C. N. (1956).
    Somatic afferent areas I and II of dog's cerebral
    cortex. J.Neurophysiol. 19: 485-499.
SOLTMAN O. (1876). Experimentalle Studien über die
    Funktionen des Grosshirns der Neugeborenen. Jahrbuch
    für Kinderheilkunde und physische Erziehung.9: 106-148.
TARCHANOFF I. (1878). Sur les centres psychomoteurs des
    animaux nouveau-nés (lapin, chien, cochon d'Inde)·Rev.
    mens.méd.chir., 2: 826.
TOWER S. S. (1940). Pyramidal lesion in the monkey.
    Brain 63: 36-90.
VONEIDA T. J. (1967). The effect of pyramidal lesions
    on the performance of a conditioned avoidance response
    in cats. Expl.Neurol. 19: 483-493.
WEED L. H. and LANGWORTHY O. R. (1926). Physiological
    study of cortical motor areas in young kittens and in
    adult cats. Contr.Embryol., 17: 89-106.
WELKER W. I., BENJAMIN R. M., MILES R. C. and WOOLSEY C.
    N. (1957). Motor effects of stimulation of cerebral
    cortex of squirrel monkey (Saimiri sciureus), J.Neuro-
    physiol. 20: 347-364.
WIESENDANGER M. (1969). The pyramidal tract. Recent in-
    vestigation on its morphology and function. Ergebn.
    Physiol. 61: 72-136.
WOOLSEY C. N., SETTLAGE P. H., MEYER D. R., SENCER W.,
    PINTO-HAMUY T. and TRAVIS A. M. (1952). Patterns of
    localization in precentral and "supplementary" motor
    areas and their relation to the concept of a premotor
    area. Res.Publ.,·Ass.Res.Nerv.Ment.Dis. 30: 238-264.
WOOLSEY C. N., GORSKA T., WETZEL A., ERICKSON T. C. and
    ALLMAN J. (1970). Patterns of localization in the
    "motor" cortex of the dog. Physiologist, 13: 348.
WOOLSEY C. N., GORSKA T., WETZEL A., ERICKSON T. C.,
    EARLS F. J. and ALLMAN J. M. (1972). Complete unilater-
    al section of the pyramidal tract at the medullary
    level in Macaca Mulatta. Brain Research, 40: 119-123.

ON THE NEUROMUSCULAR ORIGIN OF THE PHYSIOLOGICAL POSTURAL TREMOR

V. Gatev and I. Ivanov

From the Laboratory of Physiology
Research Institute of Pediatrics

Sofia, Bulgaria

It is difficult to consider the problem of the tremor origin without exactly defining what kind of movements are described by the term "tremor". If we admit that all the oscillations of the body or of parts of the body are tremor, the problem of its origin becomes very difficult, as different types of tremor would have different origins.

In this paper we consider the physiological postural tremor which may be defined as involuntary oscillations of parts of the body occurring when a normal subject voluntarily maintains a constant posture.

There are different hypotheses on the mechanisms participating in the genesis of the physiological postural tremor. The neuromuscular origin of the tremor is accepted today by many authors. According to the adherents to the alphamotoneurone hypothesis, the activation of the alphamotoneurones causes muscle microcontractions followed by tremor (Gelfand , Gurfinkel, Koz. Krinskii, Zetlin, Shik, 1964). This activation may come from supraspinal nerve centres or via the stretch reflex. The adherents to the servohypothesis, recognise only the latter mechanism (Merton, 1953 ; Halliday and Redfearn, 1956; Lippold, Redfearn and Vučo,1957). The "mechanical filter" hypothesis implies that the muscle functions as a low-pass filter that cuts off the high frequency neural discharges except those below 10 to 15 cycles per second (Marshall and Walsh, 1956). The early cerebral hypothesis explaining the tremor as an

effect of oscillating brain electrical activity (Jasper
and Andrews, 1938) has no more followers today.

Some authors claim that the physiological tremor
is not of neuromuscular origin but represents minute
oscillations arising from ballistocardiac impulses (Brumlik, 1962; Van Bushkirk and Fink, 1962; Wachs, 1964).

The present paper summarizes our experimental data
on the origin of tremor.

In the first series, we examined the influence of
the reverse loading on the hand tremor in normal adults.
The examined Subject placed his forearm on a table,
while his hand protruded from its edge and was maintain
ed voluntarily in a straight line with the forearm, the
volar part turned to the ground. A weight was attached
to the distal part of the hand by an elastic thread
passed on a pulley. In that case the weight had an anti-
gravitational effect. The Subject was instructed to
keep his hand immobile.

The tremor was measured by means of the tensometric
method, proposed by Gurfinkel,Koz and Shik (1965). The
tensometers were fastened over a flat steel spring and
the latter was fixed on the distal part of the forearm
and the proximal part of the hand. The tensometers were
connected in a bridge circuit and the measuring diagonal of the bridge was fed to the input of a tensometric
amplifier.

The electrical activity of the extensor and flexor
muscles of the hand was recorded by means of a pair of
skin electrodes (6 x 12 mm), placed 15 mm apart.

We examined the tremor and the electrical activity
of the muscles without loading, with reverse loading
equal to the hand weight, and with reverse loading
greater than the hand weight.

In the case without loading the extensor muscles
had to maintain the posture overcoming the hand weight.
Then we recorded the electrical activity in the extensor
muscles and the tremor of the hand (Fig. 1a).

In the case of reverse loading equal to the hand
weight in fact we have no actual loading. Then the
tremor amplitudes decrease and in some cases completely
disappear. The electrical activity of the muscles disappears as well (Fig. 1b).

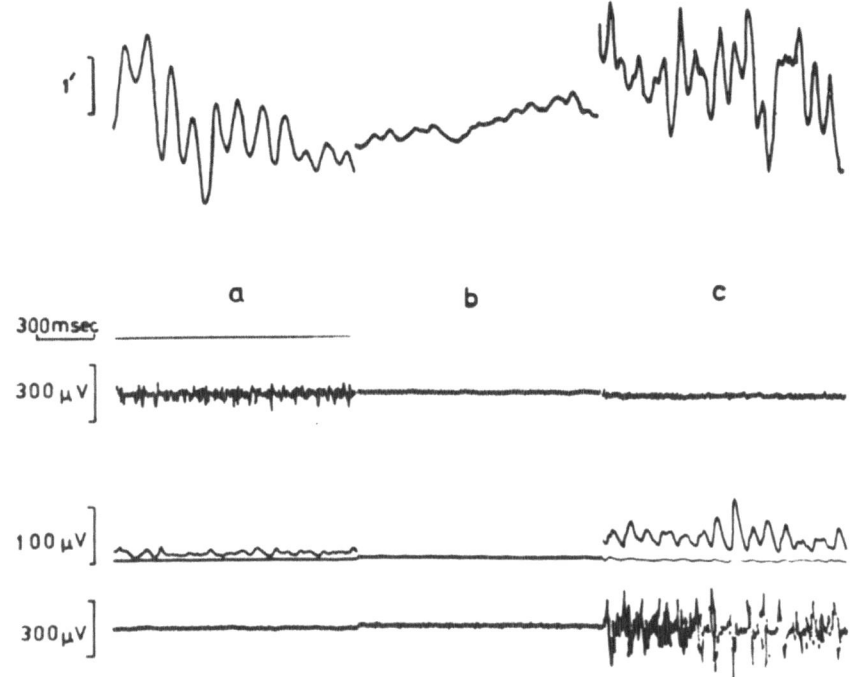

Fig. 1   Influence of reverse loading on hand tremor
          a - without loading; b - with reverse loading
          equal to hand weight; c - with reverse loading
          exceeding the hand weight with one and a half
          kilogram. First channel - tremorogram, in which
          an upward displacement corresponds to extension.
          Its amplitudes **are** calibrated in angular units;
          second - EMG of wrist-extensor; third - mean
          voltage of extensor (thick curve) and flexor
          (thin curve); fourth - EMG of wrist-flexor.

     When we applied to the reverse load equal to the
hand weight an additional weight (from 200 to 1500
grams), the tremor and the muscle activity reappeared,
but now the latter was in the flexors (Fig.1c).

     These experiments show that the postural tremor
appears and disappears with muscle activation and in-
activation. It is difficult to reconcile these findings
with the cardiac hypothesis as to the tremor origin.
Our results agree with those of Marsden, Meadows, Lange
and Watson (1969) according to whom there is no evidence
that the postural tremor is due to cardiac thrusts. The
fact the tremor and muscle activity appear and disappear
simultaneously gives solid ground for supporting the
neuromuscular origin of the postural tremor.

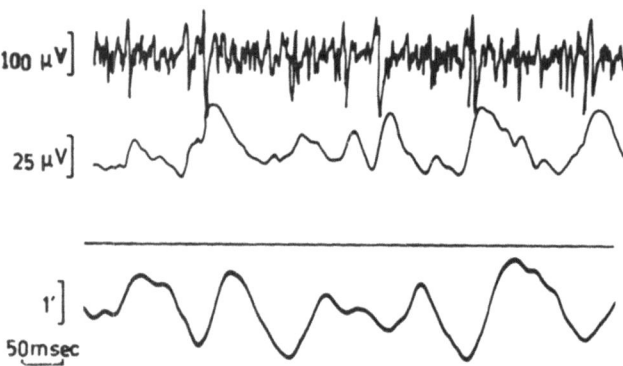

<u>Fig. 2</u>   Well expressed synphasic relations between the
         tremor and the mean voltage of the EMG. First
         channel - EMG of m.extensor digitorum; second -
         its mean voltage; third - tremor of the third
         finger.

In the next series we studied the tremor of the
third finger and the electrical activity of m.extensor
digitorum. The examined person placed his forearm and
hand on a table. The volar surface of the hand adhered
to the table, the tip of the third finger protruded
from the table edge. The tremor was recorded in the area
of the metacarpophalangeal joint in a position of slight
extension. The finger had to remain motionless. The EMG,
its mean voltage and the tremor were recorded simultaneously at 20 cm/sec.

We chose this experimental set for the following
reasons: 1. The said posture is maintained by activation
of one muscle alone, the extensor digitorum. This makes
the analysis of the relationship between EMG and tremor
easier. If the posture is maintained by several muscles
it is rather difficult to differentiate the influence of
each on the tremor oscillations. 2. The mean voltage
oscillations of the EMG, picked up by skin electrodes,
corresponds to the increase and decrease in the summary
electrical activity of the muscle. If it oscillates
synchronously with the tremor this is a solid proof for
the neuromuscular origin of the latter.

The results showed that there are time-locked relations between the tremor oscillations and the mean
voltage of the EMG. The in-phase relations were conspicuous when the EMG was synchronized with greater or

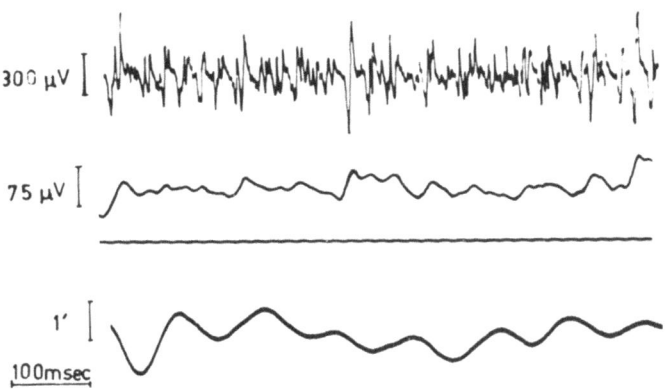

300 μV

75 μV

1'

100msec

Fig. 3   Poorly expressed synphasic relations between
the tremor and the mean voltage of the EMG.

lesser grouping of action potentials (Fig. 2). Than the
pattern of the tremor seemed to be more regular. The
phase relations were barely if at all discernible when
the EMG was asynchronous (Fig. 3). Then the pattern of
the tremor was more irregular. These findings support
the opinion as to the neuromuscular origin of the tremor.

In the next series we examined also the middle
finger tremor and the EMG of m.extensor digitorum. The
position of the finger was as in the former series, but
the fingertip was loaded with 50 grams. The aim of this
loading was to increase the synchronization of the EMG.

In these conditions we found the existence of two
distinct types of tremor (Fig. 4). One of them had
small variable amplitude, of irregular form and arhythm-
ic character. It was similar to the ordinary physiological postural tremor which may be obtained even without
loading. The second tremor pattern had larger amplitudes,
regular rhythm and form, resembling sinusoidal oscillations. In normal persons it may be recorded only after
loading.

When a regular tremor was recorded, the EMG synchronization was well expressed by grouping of action
potentials followed by silent periods (Fig. 5). The onset
of the digital flexion coincided with the silent period.
The absence of muscle activity during the silent period
made the flexion possible under the influence of the
finger weight and the loading. The flexion of the finger
extends the extensor muscle and elicits its stretch

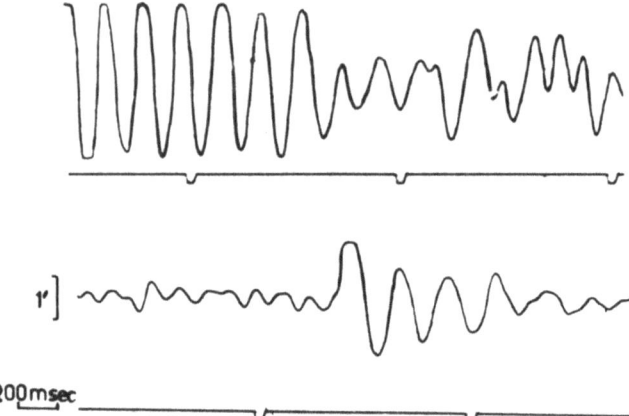

<u>Fig. 4</u>   Transition of regular tremor of the third finger
         into irregular (upper record), and of irregular
         tremor into regular (lower record).

reflex. The latter causes contraction of the muscle and
extension of the finger. In the EMG the stretch reflex
was manifested by a grouping of potentials followed by
silent periods.

     When an irregular tremor was recorded the grouping
of the action potentials was more or less marked, but

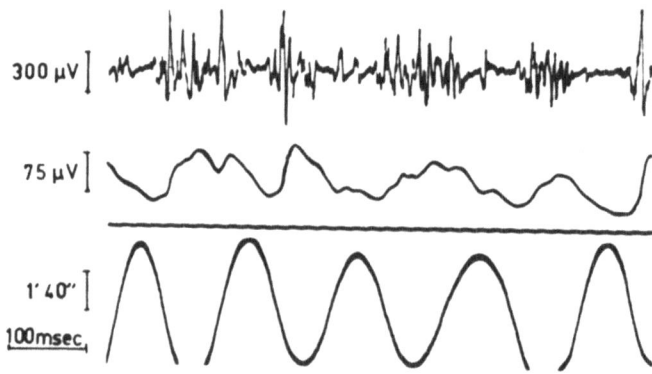

<u>Fig. 5</u>   Regular tremor. First channel - electromyogram
         of m.extensor digitorum; second channel - its
         mean voltage; third channel - tremor of the
         third finger.

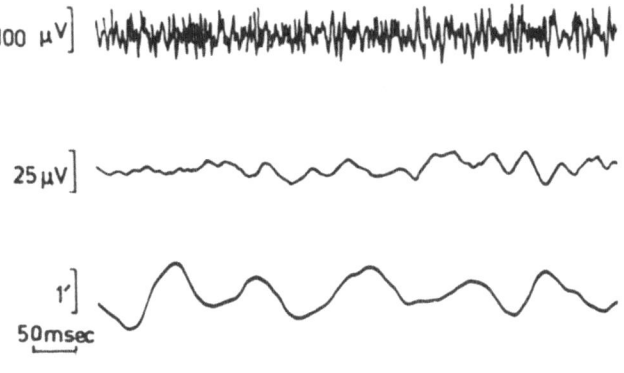

Fig. 6   Irregular tremor.

the electrical activity between the individual groups
did not disappear entirely, and the silent period was
not recorded (Fig. 6). Therefore, in this case, there
is no definite electromyographic evidence for an activation of the servomechanisms. The grouping of action
potentials without silent periods may be conceived as
an incomplete eliciting of the stretch reflex or as a
purely stochastic process resulting from supraspinal
activation of the alphamotoneurones. The latter suggestion was made by Taylor (1961) and developed by Feldman
(1964). Our further experiments were devoted to this
problem.

    We studied regular and irregular tremor patterns
of the third finger and the electrical activity of m.
extensor digitorum after procain infiltration in the
motor end-plate region. Matthews and Rushword (1957a,
1957b) found that dilute procain blocks selectively
the gamma-motor fibers without altering the transmission in the alpha-motor and the sensitive fibers. We
used five ml of an one percent procain solution, according to the method of Matthews and Rushword. The irregular tremor was obtained without loading the finger, the
regular one after loading with forty percent of the
maximal strength of m.extensor digitorum.

    Before and after the procain injection the maximal
strength of m.extensor digitorum was measured to make
sure that the integrity of the transmission in the alpha-
motor fibers was not altered. If the latter were affected the maximal muscle strength was expected to decrease.

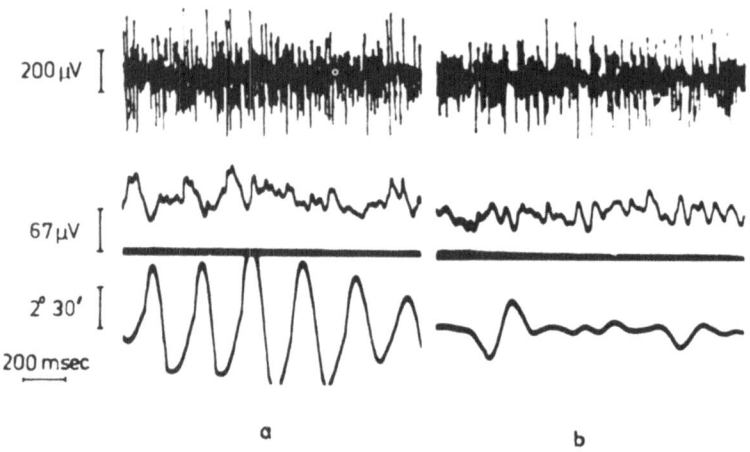

200 µV

67 µV

2° 30'

200 msec

a   b

Fig. 7   Influence of procain blockade on the regular
          tremor. a - before blockade; b - at the 15th
          minute after blockade.

     The procain interruption of the servoloop was fol-
lowed by changes in both types of tremor, better expressed in the regular one. In Fig. 7 is illustrated
the influence of the procain blockade on the regular
tremor. Its amplitude sharply diminished and in some
cases became irregular. The changes lasted from ten
to forty minutes. These results support the opinion
that in the genesis of the regular tremor the servomechanisms play an essential role.

     In Fig. 8 is illustrated the influence of dilute
procain on the irregular tremor. Its amplitude diminishes too but not so sharply. The changes lasted not more
than fifteen minutes. In some of the examined persons
no changes were found. The lesser influence of the
blockade on the irregular tremor may be explained by
the lesser participation of the servomechanism in its
genesis. A regular tremor is manifested when the finger
is loaded and the stretch reflex is elicited synchronously in all activated motor units. An irregular tremor
is obtained usually when the finger is not loaded and
the stretch reflex appears only in some motor units,
probably the units with a lower threshold of excitability. The other motor units are excited asynchronously
probably via supraspinal activation. This makes the appearance of the silent periods impossible and diminishes
the grouping of potentials, which causes the generation
of a tremor with small and irregular amplitudes.

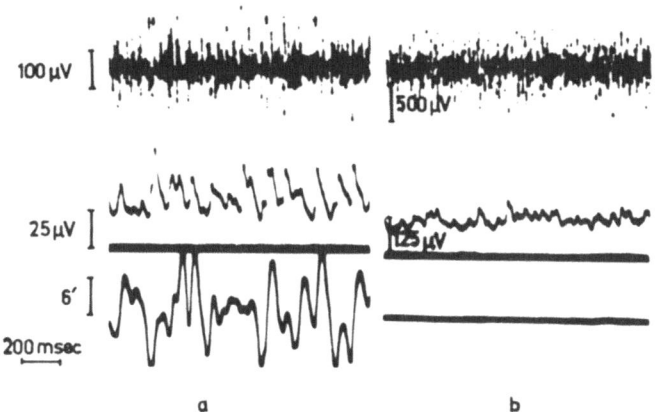

<u>Fig. 8</u>   Influence of the procain blockade on the ir-
        regular tremor:a - before blockade; b - at the
        7th minute after blockade.

    The physiological postural tremor is irregular as
a rule. The increase in neuromuscular excitability provides conditions for a more complete triggering of the
servomechanism which generates regular tremor. In our
studies the loading increases the excitability and
transforms the irregular tremor into a regular one.

    In Fig. 9 is recorded the tremor of a patient with
Parkinsonian syndrome examined without loading. The
tremor is regular. Groups of action potentials alternating with silent periods are observed in the electromyo-

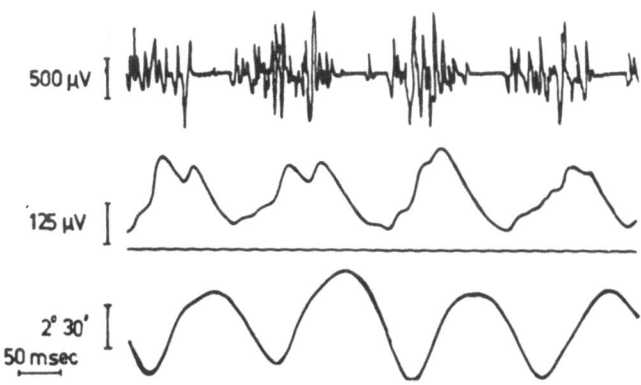

<u>Fig. 9</u>   Tremor of the third finger in a patient with
        Parkinsonian syndrome.

gram. The pattern of the tremor is similar to the regular one recorded in normal persons after loading. In
these patients the abnormally increased neuromuscular
excitability seems to be responsible for the triggering
of the total servomechanism, generating regular tremor.

In the light of these considerations we are prone
to believe that in the genesis of the physiological
postural tremor the essential role is played by the
neuromuscular activity. When the neuromuscular excitability is increased (normally or pathologically) the pattern of the tremor is determined primarily by the participation of the servomechanism. The influence of the
servomechanism decreases with the decrease of the neuromuscular excitability. Then the strength of the muscle
microcontractions, which cause tremor oscillations,
weaken and the tremor amplitudes diminish. The weaker
muscle microcontractions allow the mechanical properties
of the extremities to exert an essential effect upon the
tremor patterns, as assumed by Fox and Randall (1970).
This makes the tremor oscillations irregular and ar-
rhythmic. In these conditions the muscle may function
as a low-pass filter. When the examined part of the
body is relaxed the neuromuscular activity disappears.
Then it is possible to find the oscillations arising
from ballistocardiac impulses (Marsden et al.,1969).

In conclusion we would like to emphasize once more
that the physiological postural tremor is generated by
more than one mechanism. In some cases these may be
distinguished while in other that is impossible. Anyway,
the theories based on the assumption of only one mechanism responsible for tremor generation do not fit satis-
factorily with the experimental facts.

R E F E R E N C E S

BRUMLIK J. (1962). On the nature of normal tremor. Neuro-
    logy (Minneap.) 12: 159-179.
FELDMAN A.G. (1964). Spectrum estimation of physiologic-
    al tremor on the basis of data on work with motor
    units. Biofizika (Moskow). 9: 726-730.
FOX J.R. and RANDALL J.E. (1970). Relationship between
    forearm tremor and the biceps electromyogram. J.Appl.
    Physiol. 29: 103-108.
GELFAND I.M., GURFINKEL V.S., KOZ Y.M., KRINSKII V.I.,
    ZETLIN M.L. and SHIK M.L. (1964). Study of postural
    activity. Biofizika (Moskow). 9: 710-717.

GURFINKEL V.S., KOZ Y.M. and SHIK M.L. (1965). Control
  of posture in man. Moskow: Nauka (in Russian).
HALLIDAY A.M. and Redfearn J.W.T. (1956). An analysis
  of the frequencies of finger tremor in healthy subjects. J.Physiol.(Lond.). 134: 600-611.
JASPER H.H. and ANDREWS H.L. (1938). Brain potentials
  and voluntary muscle activity in man. J.Neurophysiol.
  1: 87-100.
LIPPOLD O.C.J., REDFEARN J.W.T. and VUČO J. (1957). The
  rhythmical activity of groups of motor units in the
  voluntary contraction of muscle. J.Physiol.(Lond.)
  137: 473-487.
MARSDEN C.D., MEADOWS J.G., LANGE G.W. and Watson R.S.
  (1969). The role of the ballistocardiac impulse in
  the genesis of physiological tremor. Brain, 92: 647-
  662.
MARSHALL J. and WALSH H.G. (1956). Physiological tremor.
  J.Neurol.Neurosurg. Psychiat. 12: 260-267.
MATTHEWS P.B.C. and RUSHWORTH G. (1957[a]). The selective
  effect of procaine on the stretch reflex and tendon
  jerk of soleus muscle when applied to its nerve.
  J.Physiol.(Lond). 135: 245-262.
MATTHEWS P.B.C. and RUSHWORTH G. (1957[b]). The relative
  sensitivity of muscle nerve fibers to procaine. J.
  Physiol.(Lond.), 135: 263-269.
MERTON P.A. (1953). Speculations on the servo control
  of movement in the spinal cord. p. 300. In Ciba Founda-
  tion Symposium, London, Churchill.
TAYLOR A. (1961). Grouping of action potentials in
  voluntary muscle. J.Physiol.(Lond.).157: 55-56.
VAN BUSHKIRK G. and FINK R. (1962). Physiologic tremor:
  an experimental study. Neurology (Minneap.) 12: 361-
  370.
WACHS H. (1964). Studies of physiologic tremor in the
  dog. Neurology (Minneap.) 14: 50-61.

ON THE SPONTANEOUS AND INDUCED BODY OSCILLATIONS

G. Gantchev, S. Dunev and N. Draganova

From the Research Institute for Work Hygiene
and Labour Protection
Sofia, Bulgaria

The body oscillations are studied in order to investigate the maintenance of the equilibrium and the
relevant factors in this respect or in the search of
new diagnostic tools in certain pathological conditions. Research in this field was initiated in the last
century with the work of Hinsdale (1887), Leitersdorfer (1897) and others, and has continued and widened
ever since. The fact that so old a problem still focus-
es such a widespread interest is primarily explained by
its particular practical value. Thus it will hardly be
an overestimation to state that investigation of space
is, to a certain extent, related to advance in the
understanding and control of the body equilibrium. The
same applies to certain branches of clinical medicine,
as neurology and oto-neurology, applied physiology and
ergonomy.

Various disciplines are concerned with investigations in the field of body equilibrium. This is mainly
due to the complexity of inter-related mechanisms which
govern the stability of the body. As it is well known,
most of the studies deal with the role of the vestibular apparatus and the visual system. Less work has been
done on the reflex mechanisms implicated in the maintenance of equilibrium. In general, the complexity of
the mechanisms, the diversity of the problems, the
specifity of the interests and the different approaches
have originated different philosophies and techniques
of investigation of the oscillations of the body. However, our task is not to make an extensive review of

the literature on this subject, but rather to present a
survey of our own work on the spontaneous and induced
oscillations of the body, with an attempt to analyze in
some detail the role of the visual system and proprioception in the maintenance of equilibrium.

As induced oscillations we shall regard only those,
resulting from an external mechanical disturbance. All
the other cases will be considered as spontaneous oscillations. Much as we are aware of the arbitrary character
and limitations of that division we have to adopt it in
order to define more sharply the field of our consideration.

We shall dwell mainly on two sets of problems:
- The role of the visual system for the maintenance of
    equilibrium
- Characteristics of induced oscillations

MATERIAL AND METHODS

One of the most sensitive and most widely used
methods of recording the body oscillations is the method
of the tensometric platform, called stabilography or
statokinesimetry. However, the very principle of the
method, as well as some practical considerations make
this technique cumbersome when one wishes to study the
response of the standing subject to a graded, mechanical
disturbance of the equilibrium. For this reason we have
elaborated a technique suitable for the investigation
of both induced and spontaneous oscillations, consisting of the following hardware:

1. A mobile platform for applying graded disturbances
to the standing subject. The platform is actuated by
means of an electro-motor and can oscillate around a
horizontal axis or make to-and-fro movements in the
ground plane. The amplitudes of these movements can be
regulated to a maximum of $\pm 6^\circ$ for the rotation and $\pm$
20 mm for the translation. The frequency range is 0.1 -
1.5 Hz.

2. Recording device. A fixed tensometric transducer
is connected by means of a string and a small constant
magnet to a metallic plate in a belt worn by the subject. In case of an unexpected pull the string and the
tensiometer are disconnected. The output of the transducer is of the order of 1 mV, the maximum tension for

a full deflexion is below 100 g. The signal from the
transducer is amplified and either recorded from CRO
tube or stored on magnetic tape for further processing.

3. Signal processing. A histogram of the body positions has been obtained with the Bruel & Kjaer apparatus
for amplitude and frequency analysis (Fig. 1).

Some minor modifications of the experimental
techniques will be described in the following chapters.

ROLE OF THE VISUAL SYSTEM FOR THE MAINTENANCE
OF EQUILIBRIUM

The influence of the visual system on the stability
of the posture has caught the interest of the early investigators of the maintenance of the equilibrium. The
first findings emphasized that the amplitude of the
oscillations of the body increases when the eyes are
closed. This increase can attain 50% (Edwards, 1946)
and even more (Latmanisova, 1931). The cause of this
effect has been sought in the interruption of the flow
of information from the outer world. Evidence in favor
of this hypothesis has been presented by Straton as
early as 1896, who found that wearing prismatic lenses
increased the body oscillations. More recently Cantrel
(1963) finds that a tachistoscopic presentation of figures decreases the oscillations in comparison to a
blank screen. Other authors. as Wapner and Witkin(1950)
report that the body oscillations decrease with an increasing complexity of the visual field.

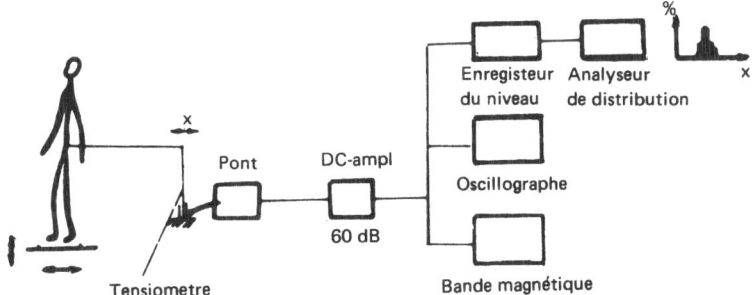

Fig. 1   Block-diagram of the experimental set up for obtaining the histogram of the position of a given
point of the body.

These findings have stimulated investigations of the effect of illumination on the body oscillations. A great part of the research in that field is due to Gurfinkel and his collaborators (Gurfinkel, Kotz and Shik, 1965; Gurfinkel and Elner, 1971).It has been found by these authors that closing the eyes and turning the light off increase the amplitude of the oscillations but the effect of the former is more pronounced. What is more, closing the eyes in darkness continues to increase slightly the oscillations. These workers explain the effect of light with conditioned experience, the level of illumination being a signal for expectancy of information. On the other hand, it has been shown (Wapner and Witkin, 1950, Witkin and Wapner, 1950) that a reduction of the information leads to an increase of the body oscillations. Litvinenkova and Hlavacka (1971) have found that there is a decrease of the amplitude of body oscillations in dark adaptation which is more marked in closing the eyes. Though no satisfactory explanation of this phenomenon can be offered , it has been argued that there is some disturbance of the light-conditioned reflexes during dark adaptation or that some effect could be played by the eye movements (Litvinenkova and Baron, 1968). The visual information seems to act as a negative feedback in the maintenance of body equilibrium. Thus Travis (1944) has shown that keeping balance on an unstable platform is facilitated when there is visual feedback about the position of the body. Similar data are presented by Hlavacka and Litvinenkova (1972), according to whom stability was increased when the subject was allowed to observe his oscillations on a screen.

The investigations of the role of the visual information in the maintenance of the equilibrium has raised intriguing questions on the importance of eye movements, especially since it has been observed that the body oscillations increase when the subject looks at moving objects. Wapner and Witkin (1950) report that the body stability is reduced when one stares at a cube, irregularly oscillating in the dark, Edwards (1943,1946) finds that the body oscillations are increased when observing a 15° sway of a pendulum. These and other data suggest that the movements of the eyes play a definite role in the control of equilibrium. This problem is discussed in detail by Baron (1951, 1963).

Our own attempts to analyze the role of the visual information and eye movements in the maintenance of equilibrium are described below.

The oscillations of the body and its position were recorded in healthy subjects, first two minutes eyes closed, then two minutes eyes open. The duration of the experiment seemed a reasonable compromise between the wish to avoid fatigue and the need to have a sufficient number of waves in order to compute the histogram of the body position. Gurfinkel et al. (1965) have shown that there are no signs of fatigue in a two minute record.

RESULTS

a) Effect of eyes closure on the amplitude of the oscillations and on the position of the body.

It has been confirmed in 20 Subjects that the amplitudes increase when the eyes were closed.However a closer analysis showed that this increase interests mainly the oscillations in the medium amplitude range. The slower, higher oscillations also increase as a rule, but there are cases in which the opposite effect can be observed (Fig. 2).

It was more interesting to note the effect on the body position. In 18 from our 20 Subjects we found a forward shift in closing the eyes. This shift was variously expressed: 5 mm in the average but could attain 10 mm and more in some subjects (Gantchev, Koitcheva, Draganova and Gantcheva, 1971). These findings are illustrated in the following two records (Figs.2 and 3). We can see not only an increase of the amplitudes of the oscillations in closing of the eyes, but also a bias of the base   expressing the forward shift of the body. The histograms also show that during the two minute record with eyes closed, the body has stayed longer frontally to the base line than when the eyes were open (Fig. 4). This phenomenon has also been observed by other authors. Thus on Fig.5, reprinted from Gurfinkel et al.(1965) we find that the oscillations of

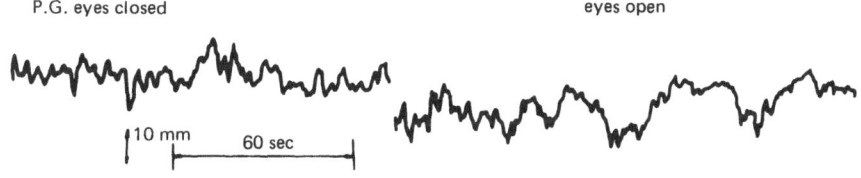

P.G. eyes closed   eyes open

10 mm   60 sec

Fig. 2   Record of the body oscillations (Subject P.G.) eyes open and eyes closed. With eyes closed the amplitudes decrease in contrary of the common rule.

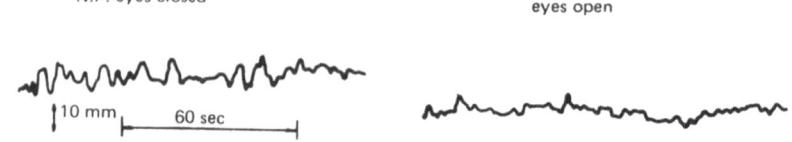

N.P. eyes closed   eyes open

Fig. 3   Record of the body oscillations (Subject N.P.)
          eyes open and eyes closed. The 5-10 mm forward
          inclination of the body when the eyes are clos-
          ed is expressed by an upward shift of the base
          line.

the centre of gravity with eyes closed are biased forwards in respect to the base line.

     Two new series of experiments were set up in order
to analyze this phenomenon. In the first one ten Subjects were instructed to open and close the eyes succes-
sively during two minutes, then, after a pause, the
task was repeated. The analysis of the records has shown

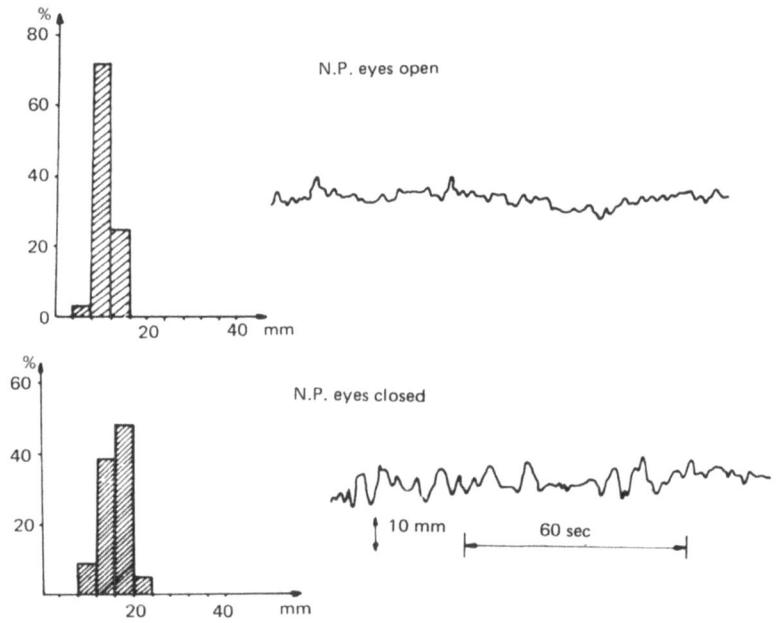

Fig. 4   The histogram of the body position in the "eyes
          closed" position is characterized by a shift
          to the right, corresponding to the forward in-
          clination and a larger dispersion.

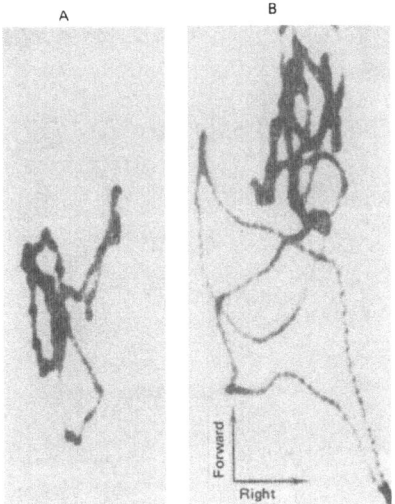

Fig. 5   Vectograms of a body point: a) eyes open, b)
         eyes closed.

that the first response to closing the eyes is a
rapid inclination forwards. Some time later there is a
more or less evident slower continuing of the inclination. The reverse phenomenon is observed when the eyes
are opened. It can therefore be argued that the response of the body to opening or closing of the eyes
contains a rapid early and a slower later component,
but this phenomenon is not always clear.

       In order to assess the possible influence of the
eyes position, knowing that when the eyes are closed
the eye-balls rotate upwards, we asked another series
of 14 Subjects to stand on the platform for two minutes,
the gaze parallel to the ground, then to shift the eyes
to the ceiling for another two minutes without moving
the head. In 50% of our Subjects this upward rotation
of the eye-balls was followed by a slight or more marked forward inclination of the body, with some increase
of the amplitude of the oscillations.

       b) Effect of the eye-ball position and the eye
movements on the stability of the body.
       The role of the tonic contractions of the eye musc-
les was investigated in a series of 20 Subjects placed
in front of a white screen, at a distance of 1.5 m. They
were instructed to look at a horizontal plane (2 min)
then upwards (2 min) and then downwards (2 min). The
position of the head was controlled visually by the ex-

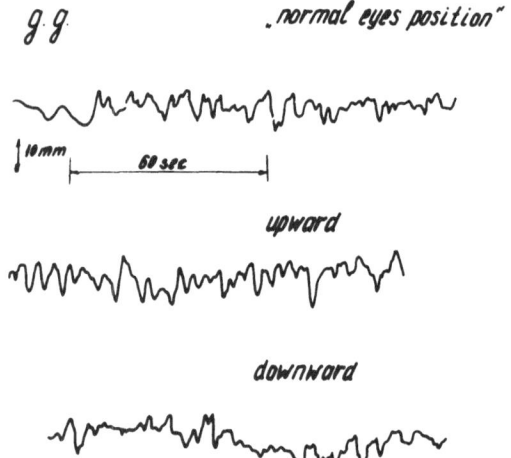

Fig. 6   Records of the body oscillations with different fixation of the gaze.

perimenter. It was found as a rule, that the upward gaze provoked an increase of the amplitude of the body oscillations. When the gaze was directed downwards the amplitude decreased, in some Subjects it was even lower than in the control, horizontal position of the eyeballs. These results are illustrated on Fig.6.

The role of the eye movements was investigated by means of induced optokinetic nystagmus. A rotating translucent, internally illuminated drum was placed 40 cm in front of the Subject. The drum displayed a black-and-white checkerboard pattern. The size of the squares was 1 cm. The velocity of rotation was variable between 1.4°/sec to 143.8°/sec. Control records were taken before and after the induced nystagmus.

The obtained results are illustrated by the two stabilograms on Figs 7 and 8. It is seen that during optokinetic nystagmus there is a very marked - more than twice-increase of the body oscillations. No correlation was found with the speed of rotation although the latter affects the rapidity of the slow component of the nystagmus (Gantchev et al.,1971; Koitcheva and Gantchev, 1972).

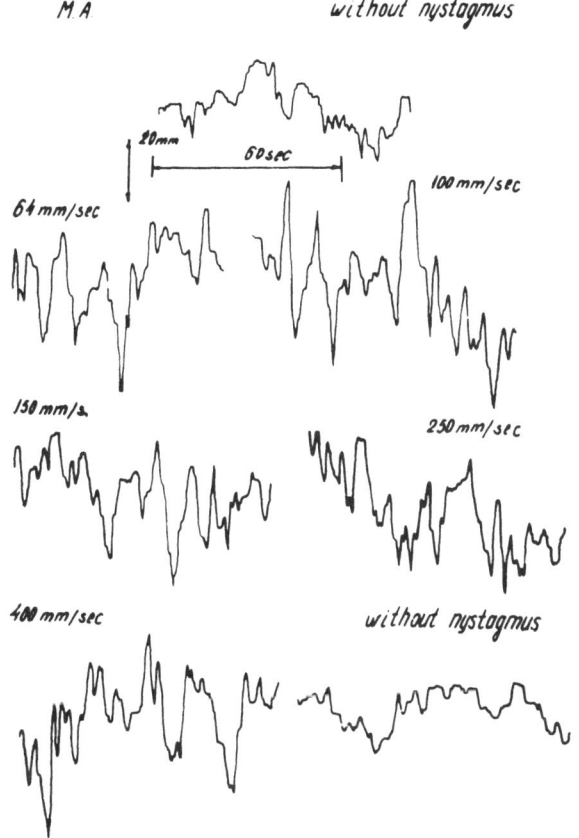

Fig. 7   Body oscillations (Subject St.D.) in induced
optokinetic nystagmus   at different speeds of
the black-and-white checkerboard pattern.

DISCUSSION

The first intriguing phenomenon is the forward inclination of the body when the eyes are closed, with its
rapid and slow components. This is a complex reaction of
redistribution of the muscular tonus. It could be partly
triggered by the upward rotation of the eyes which is
contingent to the closure of the lids. We have seen in
our experiments that a voluntary upward fixation of the
gase was sufficient only in several numbers of cases, to
provoke the forward inclination. That's why this assumption needs more evidences. Biologically, the forward inclination can be conceived as a defense reaction against
a possible fall when the eyes are closed. In that case
falling forwards could be preferable as the arms can
protect the body and the face.

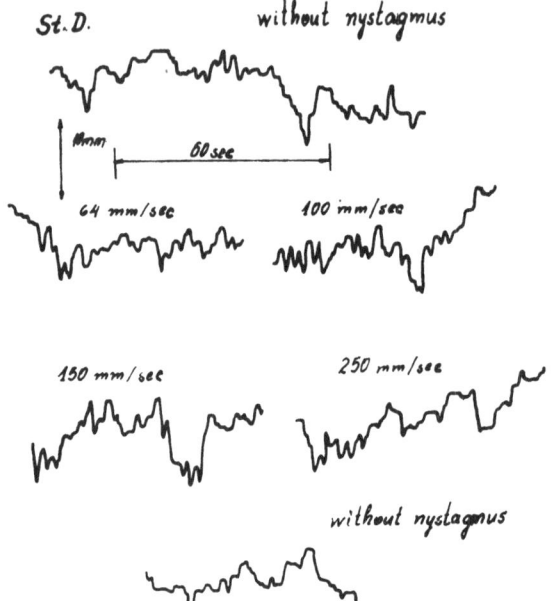

<u>Fig. 8</u>   Body oscillations (Subject M.A.). The conditions
         as in Fig. 7.

    In the last series of experiments it has been found
that the eye movements played a definite role in the
control of equilibrium. It was also shown that an upward
fixation of the gaze decreases the stability of the body
whereas a downward fixation improves it. An explanation
of these opposite effects could be sought in the following considerations:

    a) The mechanics of the upward and downward eye
detections are different. The upward fixation causes
greater muscular strain as the superior oblique muscle
is smaller than the inferior oblique.

    b) The central regulation of these two movements is
different. It has been found in cats that the medial
part of the superior collicle was primarily concerned
with upward gaze while the lateral part controls the
downward movements. Similar relations are supposed in
man.

    c) It could be also argued that the improvement of
stability when looking downwards is due to a life-long
training to work in these conditions of vision. This
behavioural pattern could form the basis of a natural
conditioned mechanism which improves stability when the
gaze descends bellow the horizontal plane. The movements

of the head would also probably be involved in this hypothetical mechanism.

The other problem is whether the eye movements or
the tonic fixation of the eye-balls are in themselves
responsible for the effects on the control of equilibrium
or the response is associated with changes in visual information. It is difficult at present to find a satisfactory answer to that question, but we presume that in
certain conditions the specific eye muscle activity
could trigger alone the control mechanism of equilibrium.
Part of our assumptions is based on the results with
optokinetic nystagmus which elicits a marked deterioration of stability. We have shown in a previous work(Koitcheva and Gantchev,1972) that with an angular velocity
of the stimulus of the order of 10-15° p.sec., these is
a synchronization between the stimulus and the slow component of the optokinetic nystagmus. In these conditions, we have a retinal fixation of the image during
90% of the time. The perception of the object will be
disturbed only during the rapid phase of the nystagmus.
At higher speeds there is no synchronization. Nevertheless the troubles of stability are the same over all
the range of stimulus speeds. This reasoning leads us
to assume that the eye movements in themselves can play
role in disturbing the stability of the body.

The question of the inter-relations between visual
information and eye movements in producing this effect
needs further investigation.

INDUCED OSCILLATIONS OF THE BODY

In recent years the system approach which proved
so fruitful in technology has been widely used for the
description and analysis of biological systems. We have
attempted to follow that line in a quantitative investigation of the input-output relations of the system responsible for the control of equilibrium. By means of a
mobile platform (see Material and Methods) on which the
Subject is standing, we applied graded disturbances and
studied the body response by recording the oscillations
at the level of the centre of gravity.

Ten volunteers served as Subjects for this experiment. Three others were examined three times. They were
instructed to step on the mobile platform and try to
maintain the upright posture. Two kinds of disturbances
of the system were applied:

a) The plat orm oscillates around a horizontal axis corresponding to the axis of the talo-crural joint. The amplitude of the oscillations was fixed (6°) and the frequencies were as above.

b) An to-and-fro oscillation in the horizontal plane. The amplitude of this oscillation was 4 cm, the range of frequencies applied was 0.14, 0.22, 0.33, 0.43, 0.53, 0.60, 1.25 cpsec.

We recorded the angular excursions of the talo-crural joint by means of a potentiometer and the EMG of the anterior tibialis muscle, the medial head of the gastrocnemius and the soleus.

RESULTS

a) Amplitude and phase effects elicited by angular sinusoidal displacement of the platform.
All the Subjects showed similar behaviour during rotational oscillations of the platform. The oscillations of the body are maximal at the lower frequencies of the platform: 0.14 and 0.22 cpsec. When the frequency increases to 0.68 cpsec the body oscillations are reduced and at the highest frequency - 1.25 cpsec, they become irregular and rather similar to the spontaneous body oscillations. At the same time the amplitude of the talo-crural excursions increases with the increase of the induced frequency (Fig. 9). An effect of training is easily detected. It consists of a reduction of the amplitude of the body oscillations at lower frequencies.

A certain phase lag between the oscillations of the platform and the oscillations of the body could be observed in all our cases. This phase lag was less evident at the higher frequencies. We cannot at this time present exact quantitative data on these phase relations and hope to be able to reinvestigate the problem by means of averaging techniques.

b) Amplitude and phase effects elicited by horizontal sinusoidal displacements of the platform.

The amplitude and phase effects of the horizontal displacements or the platform are roughly similar to those observed in the case of angular displacements. The amplitude of the body oscillations decreases as the frequency of the displacements augments. The excursions of the talo-crural joint are modified in the opposite sense. When the amplitudes of the body oscillations are

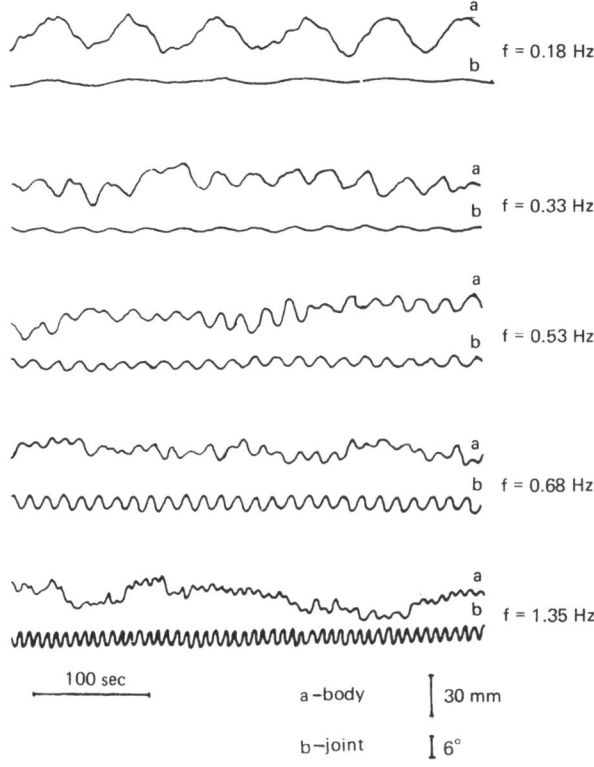

a
f = 0.18 Hz
b

a
f = 0.33 Hz
b

a
f = 0.53 Hz
b

a
f = 0.68 Hz
b

a
f = 1.35 Hz
b

100 sec

a –body   30 mm

b –joint   6°

Fig. 9.   Oscillations induced in a Subject standing on
a platform, oscillating at different frequencies around a horizontal axis. The upper record in each pair represents the oscillations
of the body, the lower one - those of the
talocrural joint.

smaller, the angular excursions of the talo-crural joint
are greater. These results are illustrated on Fig. 10.

DISCUSSION

We can not, at this stage, propose a satisfactory
global explanation of all the obtained results as it
seems that the complex neuro-regulations are complemented by no less important biomechanical factors. We shall
therefore suggest only some preliminary considerations.

Obviously, it appears from our data that the main
control of the equilibrium is exerted through various
reflex mechanisms. Undoubtedly the vestibular apparatus

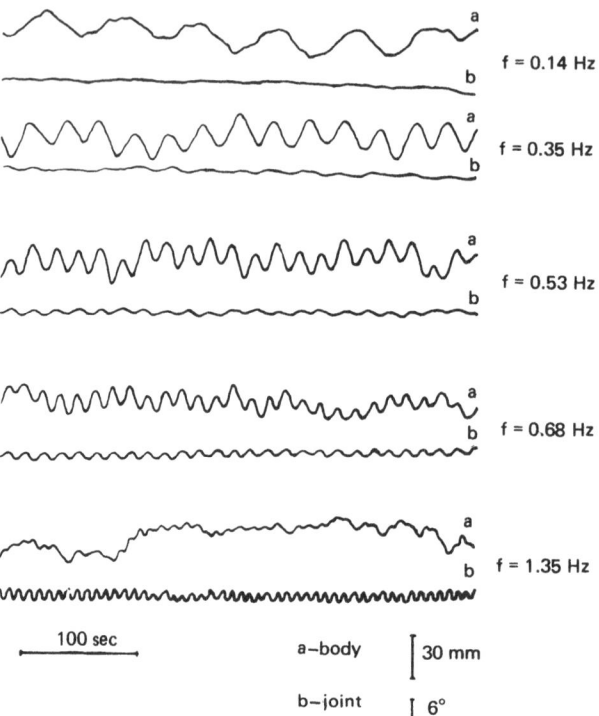

Fig. 10   Same as in Fig.9, except that the platform
           moves to-and-fro in a horizontal plane.

plays an important role for the maintenance of equilibrium in our experiments. However, vestibular control
seems to predominate in the lower frequencies of the
induced oscillations when their amplitude attains 3-4
cm, or even more. In these cases the inclination of the
body can be of the order of 2° and fall in the range
of the threshold pr slightly supra-threshold stimuli for
the vestibular apparatus. In the low frequency range
(up to 0.20 cpsec) the angular excursions of the talo-
crural joints are minimal. If that joint was mechanical-
ly following the oscillations of the platform the triceps muscle would have been elongated with a speed of
0.4-0.65 mm/sec. Actually, the computed values are 5 to
10 times lower. Consequently we can suppose that the
stretch reflex could not play a very effective role in
the control of equilibrium as the applied stimulus is
most probably subthreshold.

When the frequency of the platform is increased,
the elongation of the muscles and its first derivative
in time increase too.For the different frequencies the

speed of elongation ranges from 1 to 3.75 mm/sec. In this way the efficiency of the peripheral feedback mechanisms increases and the tracking of the platform is improved.

Another factor which could be invoked to explain the amelioration of the mechanisms of equilibrium is the pattern of activity in the antagonist muscles of the leg.

It has been found that in the low frequency range the inclinations of the body affect mainly the triceps muscle. However when the frequency of the platform increases above 0.5 cpsec, we can observe an alternating activity in the triceps muscle and in the tibialis anterior muscle. As we mentioned above the following of the platform excursions by the talo-crural joint is improved in this frequency range.

REFERENCES

BARON J.-B. (1951). Relation entre les muscles moteurs oculaires, les nageoires et l'équilibre des poissons. C.R.Acad.Sc. 231: 1087-1088.

BARON J.-B. (1963). Les troubles oculomoteurs, origine des déséquilibres du syndrome subjectif post-commotionnel. In: Proc.of the XIV Int.Congr.on Occup.Health. Madrid.

CANTREL R.P. (1963). Body balance activity and perception. Perception and Motor Skills. 17: 431-437.

EDWARDS A.S. (1943). Factors tending to decrease the steadiness of the body at rest. Am.J.Psychol. 56: 589-602.

EDWARDS A.S. (1946). Body sway and vision. J.exp.Psychol., 36: 526-535.

GANTCHEV G.N., DRAGANOVA N. and DUNEV S. (1972). The role of visual information and ocular movements for the maintenance of body equilibrium. Agressologie, 13, B: 55-61.

GANTCHEV,G., KOITCHEVA V., DRAGANOVA N. and GANTCHEVA P. (1971). Study on the involuntary movements of the eyes. In: Visual Information Processing and Control of Motor Activity, Intern.Symp., Sofia 1969, 248-258; Sofia: Publ.Bulg.Acad.Sci.

GURFINKEL V.S., KOTZ J.M. and SHICK M.L. (1965). Regulacia pozy celoveka (In Russian). Moscow, Nauka.

GURFINKEL V.S. and ELNER A.M. (1971). Zritelnij kontrol v regulacia ravnovesija. Visual Information Processing and Control of Motor Activity. Intern.Symp.,Sofia 1969: 331-335,Sofia; Publ.Bulg.Acad.Sci.

HINSDALE G. (1887). The station of man considered physiologically and clinically. Amer.J.Med.Sci., 93: 478-492.

HLAVACKA F. and LITVINENKOVA V. (1972). Visual information and control of the upright posture in man. Visual Information Processing and Control of Motor Activity. Intern.Symp.Sofia 1969: 337-341; Sofia, Publ.Bulg. Acad.Sci.

KOITCHEVA V. and GANTCHEV G. (1972). Nekotorie harakteristiki optokineticeskogo nistagma v raznich usloviach ego vozniknovenija.- Abstracts of the II Int.Symp.on Motor Control, (In Russian), Varna, 1972: 28.

LATMANISOVA L.V. (1931). Rezultati razrabotki kefalograficeskij zapisej, Tr.Leningrad.Inst.po izuceniju prof.zabol. (In Russian). 5: 163-169.

LEITERSDORFER (1897). Das militärische Traening, Stuttgart. After Gurfinkel V.S., Kotz J.M., Shik M.L. (1965). Regulacia pozy celoveka, p.31, Moscow,Nauka.

LITVINENKOVA V. and BARON J.B. (1968). Variations de la régulation posturale en fonction des informations visuelles et oculomotrices. C.R.Soc.Biol.Paris, 162: 1294.

LITVINENKOVA V. and HLAVACKA F. (1971). Visual information and regulation of motion activity of man during dark adaptation. Visual information.- Tr.Leningr.Inst. po Izuc.Prof.Zabol.,1969: 343-347.

STRATTON G.M. (1896). Some preliminary experiments on vision without inversion of the retinal image. Physiol. Rev., 3:611. After Gurfinkel V.S., Kotz J.M. Shik M.L. (1965). Regulacia pozy celoveka, p.177, Moscow.

TRAVIS R.C. (1944). A new stabilometer for measuring dynamic equilibrium in the standing position. J.exp. Psychol.,63: 385-408.

WAPNER S. and WITKIN H.A. (1950). The role of visual factors in the maintenance of body-balance. Amer.J. Psychol., 63: 385-408.

WITKIN H.A. and WAPNER S. (1950). Visual factors in the maintenance of upright posture. Amer.J.Psychol., 63: 31-50.

MUSCLE STIFFNESS AND MOTOR CONTROL - FORCES IN THE ANKLE DURING LOCOMOTION AND STANDING

Sten Grillner

From the Department of Physiology, University
of Göteborg
Göteborg, Sweden

INTRODUCTION

In order to have any idea of how CNS controls movements, we must know the general properties of the motor,
it is set to control and what is required from this
motor under normal as well as extreme conditions. We
must know how sluggish the muscles are and what forces
they can and must develop at different joint angles. We
must further know the time course of the movement we are
studying under normal and extreme conditions to be able
to evaluate if the time available permits reflex adjustments or correcting signals from higher structures during the course of the movement. This kind of data is
relatively simple to obtain, without them any discussion
of results related to the neural control of movement can
only end up in rather loose speculations.

This presentation seeks to answer some of these
questions. I have chosen the ankle of the cat as a model,
because muscles, motor units, receptors and the central
control of α- and γ- motoneurones to the ankle extensors
have been investigated in some detail (see Granit,1970),
nevertheless the motor control of the ankle joint has
not been considered as a whole. The presentation brings
out the significance of the inherent muscle stiffness
for any kind of "load compensation" (see also Rack,1970)
and at the same time it is shown that a reflex load compensation is virtually impossible during fast movements
since at the time the reflexly induced tension will

build up, the movement has already proceeded into another
phase. The force development during locomotion is calculated and the resulting length changes are discussed in
relation to muscle properties and possible reflex mechanisms, and the interaction between reflex control and inherent muscle properties is considered in particular for
the tonic stretch reflex as the best known example.

Recent studies have shown that the different ankle
extensors (the gastrocnemius, soleus and plantaris) are
more versatile than previously believed. Thus all the
muscles take part in locomotion, including the soleus
which is often considered as a postural muscle. Wetzel,
Gerlach, Stern and Hannapel (1972) looked behaviourally
on the role of different ankle extensors after having
denervated some of the extensors. In preparations with
only the gastrocnemius intact no clear deficit was seen,
whereas some deficit was observed with only soleus and
plantaris intact, but the ankle still participated ef-
ficiently during locomotion and posture as well as jumping. Similar results for the soleus have been obtained
with EMG recordings (Goslow, Reinking and Stuart,1972;
Gambarian, Orlovski, Protopopova, Severin and Shik,1971).
The motor units appear to be active in a higher frequency
range during locomotion than posture (Severin, Shik and
Orlovski,1967).

The Ankle Joint during Standing
        It thus seems meaningful to choose the ankle joint
for an analysis of biomechanical events and requirements.
At first (Fig. 1) we will consider what forces must be
developed by the ankle extensors during standing as the
angle of the ankle (A) and the angle of the foot to the
mechanical axis (α) change. The mechanical axis is
chosen as a vertical live running through the hip and
the footpads (see Fig. 1 A). The required torque at the
ankle joint depends on the distance from the ankle pivot
to the mechanical axis (h) and the load (F_V) applied
along the axis. The required force (F_M) that must be
developed by the ankle extensors to counteract any given
load is given by the equation below (see legend to Fig.1
and Grillner,1972), which is based on ordinary mechanical
and trigonometrical calculations.

$$F_M = F_V \cdot \frac{a}{b} \cdot \sin \alpha \sqrt{\frac{m^2 + b^2 - 2mb \cdot \cos(180-A)}{m \cdot \sin(180-A)}}$$

        The graph of Fig. 1 B, C is calculated with a load of
600 g on the cat, i.e. what one hindlimb carries normally

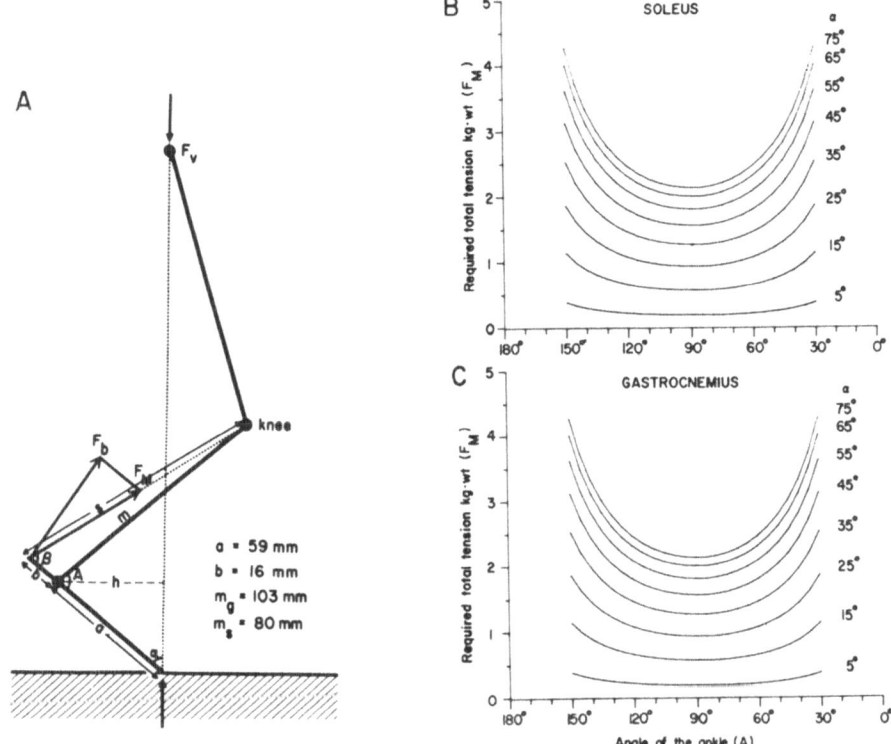

<u>Fig. 1</u>   The required force in the ankle extensors during
standing. A shows a schematical representation
of the hindlimb of a cat. The load (F_v) is applied along a vertical axis running through the
hip and the "footpads". The distance between
the ankle pivot and the mechanical axis is h_o .
The length of different bone segments (a, b)
and the distance from the muscle origin to the
ankle pivot (m) is indicated in the graph. B
and C are calculated from the eq.given in the
text, the force required at any given ankle of
the ankle (A) is plotted in B and C for different values of α i.e. the angle between the
metatarsal bones and the mechanical axis. B and
C are calculated as if the soleus or gastrocnemius should carry the entire load on the limb

(cf.Manter, 1938). The values for different angles of
the ankle (A) and different angles of the metatarsal bones
to the mechanical axis (α), are given. The calculations
are performed as if the soleus or alternatively gastrocnemius was alone responsible for the force development.

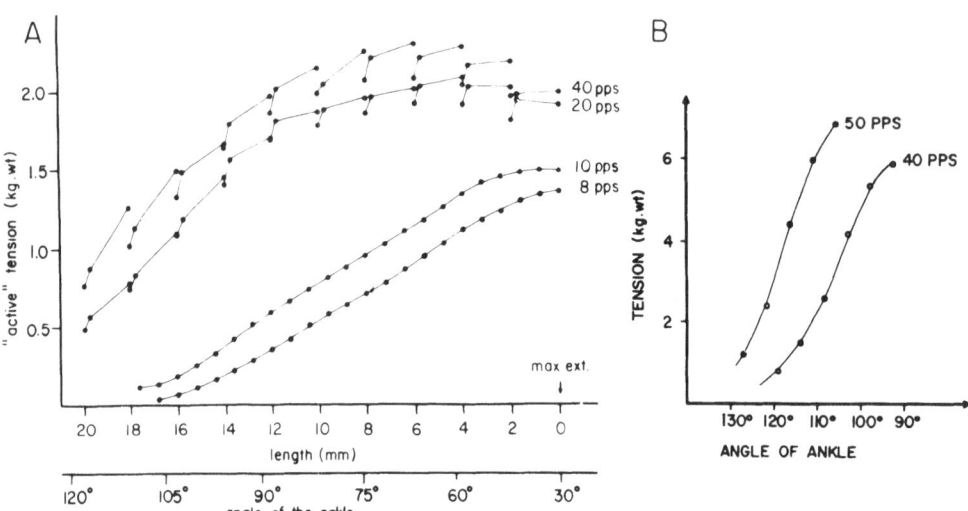

Fig. 2   Length-tension graphs of soleus and the lateral
          gastrocnemius stimulated with distributed stimula-
          tion during slow extension of the muscles. The
          ventral roots supplying the muscles were sub-
          divided in five parts; each was stimulated at a
          certain frequency but the point of stimulation
          for each part was distributed in relation to the
          other parts (see Rack and Westbury, 1969). The
          mean frequency is given at the right of each
          curve. A: soleus m., B: gastrocnemius m. at dif-
          ferent rates of activity. Ordinate: active ten-
          sion, i.e. the tension contributed by passive
          muscle properties has been subtracted from the
          total tension; the abscissa: joint angle or
          length from max.extension. Lengthening rate 0.8
          mm/sec

Ankle angles between 80° - 125° require the lowest muscle
force. This range is in fact used during standing (110°)
(Goslow et al.,1972) and during locomotion (130° - 80°)
(Engberg and Lundberg,1969). Outside this range the
force requirement increases steeply in both directions.
It is of course not unexpected to find that the most
economical point is used during ordinary locomotion and
posture although the range outside this can be used during crouching or jumping.

      If the load on the limb will increase, the joints
will flex, since the muscle force is not adequate to
counteract this load. As the limb flexes (A becomes
smaller), the required muscle force will apparently increase sharply up to the maximal muscle length(Fig. 1).

If the muscle at a given level of activity developed the
same force at any muscle length between 120° - 30°, any
lengthening of the muscle would result in a progressively
increased demand for force, a kind of "run away" would
occur. This would seem as a very unsecure system, without stability. Fortunately, the muscle does not behave
as a linear motor, and in fact the force increases sharply with increasing muscle length (Fig. 2). At low motor
unit frequencies the tension is rather low at joint
angles of 100° - 120°, but increases progressively up to
a maximal extension. At higher frequencies as typically
used in locomotion (Severin et al.,1967) the tension output is substantial also at 100° - 120°, but reaches a
ceiling at an angle of 70° - 80° and does not increase
further. Hence any increase in muscle length will result
in a marked increase in muscle force, i.e. the muscle
has a large stiffness, in the length range used in locomotion and posture.

The forces given in Fig. 2 are only that part produced by active contraction. In fact fasciae and other
connective tissue acting as parallel elastic elements
(Fig. 3) and virtually no tension at 100° - 120° but
below 90°, the passive force increases drastically to
several kg.wt.(see Grillner, 1972 and Fig. 3). How
large this value is, depends to a large extent on the
knee joint angle, mainly due to the fact that the gastrocnemius originates from the femur and has a very dense
fascia (see legend of Fig. 3). It is apparent that the
muscle force developed by purely passive factors can be
quite significant and will aid in counteracting the increased force requirement at higher muscle lengths
particularly if the knee is extended (compare the required increase of force in Fig. 1).

In the graph of Fig. 1 the vertical load on the
limb is 600 g. At a joint angle of 115° and an angle α
of 15° (mechanical axis to the metatarsal bones) the
force required is 750 g. If now an increased load of
100 g, i.e. up to 700 g, is gradually applied to the
limb the force necessary to counteract this value (850
g.wt) can be obtained by increasing α with 1° and de-
creasing the ankle angle with 1.5^o, provided that the
stiffness of the muscle is the same as that of the lateral gastrocnemius muscle in Fig. 2 B (see Grillner,1972).

From these considerations it is clear that the
muscle even without any reflex control can counteract
changes in load and must be a significant factor in the

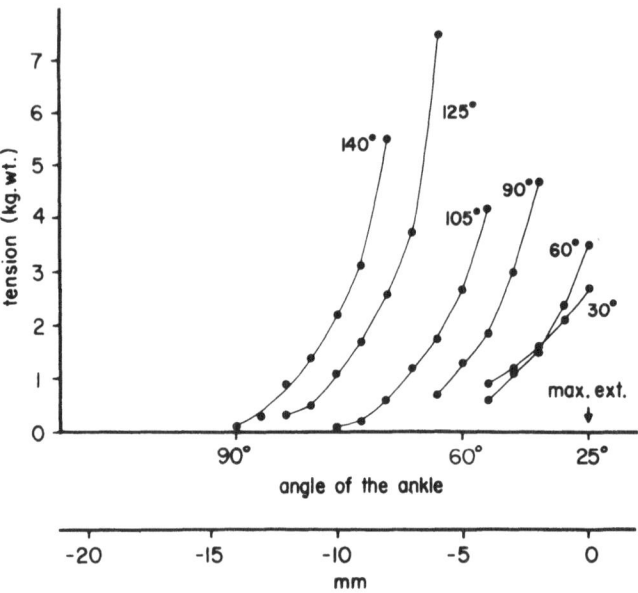

<u>Fig. 3</u>   The passive forces in the ankle joint at dif-
ferent joint angles in knee and ankle. The
ordinate shows the tension in Achilles tendon
at different angles of the ankle (abscissa). At
the right of the different curves is indicated
at what knee joint angle the values were obtained. The tension was measured by a strain-gauge
in series with the tendon; the working range and
ankle joint angles were measured accurately before disconnecting the tip of the calcaneus from
the foot. The tibia was fixed rigidly and independently of the femur; the latter fixation
was movable and allowed rapid changes of the
knee-joint angle. The length of the muscles
(corresponding to the actual ankle angle) was
modified by means of a manipulator which had an
accuracy of 0.002 mm. In order to assess the
real value of the passive forces, only the bone
insertion of the Achilles tendon was separated
from the calcaneus and no other dissection
whatsoever was performed . This is in contrast
to most experiments in which the muscles are
carefully dissected free. The curve obtained
with a knee joint angle of 30° is not parallel
to the other curves, because the muscles on the
back of the thigh are in mechanical contact with
the ankle extensors due to the marked knee flexion. This effect is somewhat increased at this
knee joint angle due to the fixation arrangement
of femur

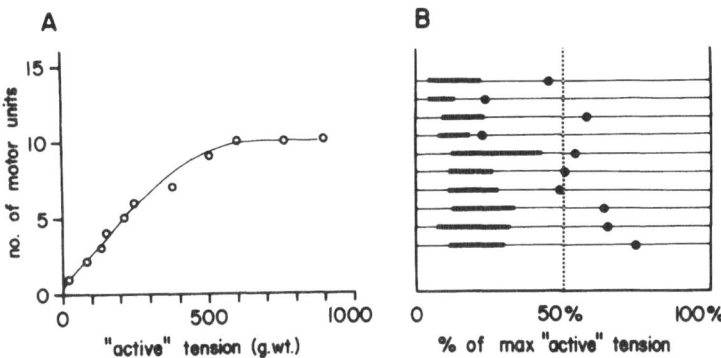

<u>Fig. 4</u>   Recruitment of motor units in the tonic stretch
           reflex of soleus m. during slow extension at
           constant velocity (decerebrate preparation).
           A: number of motor units recruited at different
           active tensions in the stretch reflex (passive
           forces subtracted). The total sample is 10 motor
           units obtained by simultaneous recording with
           three electrodes on, or in the soleus muscle,
           and thus with all elements in the stretch reflex
           intact as e.g. the ventral roots. B summarizes
           the same type of finding for 10 experiments;
           each line indicates one experiment. The left
           edge of the bar on each line indicated at what
           tension 25% of the motor units have been recruit-
           ed, the right edge when 75% and the dot when
           100% of the motor units have been recruited.
           Clearly the majority of the motor units are re-
           cruited at a tension around 30-40% of the active
           tension at maximal extension of the muscle
           (Grillner and Udo,1971 b)

length range used during standing and locomotion. If that
was not the case the biomechanical conditions in the ankle
would be very unstable. That some load compensation must
actually occur in the muscle is also indicated by the
fact that deafferented animals can stand and walk around
with ease with not too much abnormalities in their motor
performance (Taub and Berman,1968), which would otherwise be highly unlikely in view of the data of Fig. 1.

      Interaction between Reflex Mechanisms and Muscle
Properties in the Tonic Stretch Reflex

      The tonic stretch reflex in the soleus muscle has
a threshold of around 90° in the ankle and the tension
increases up to 30° (cf.Matthews,1959, Granit,1958).

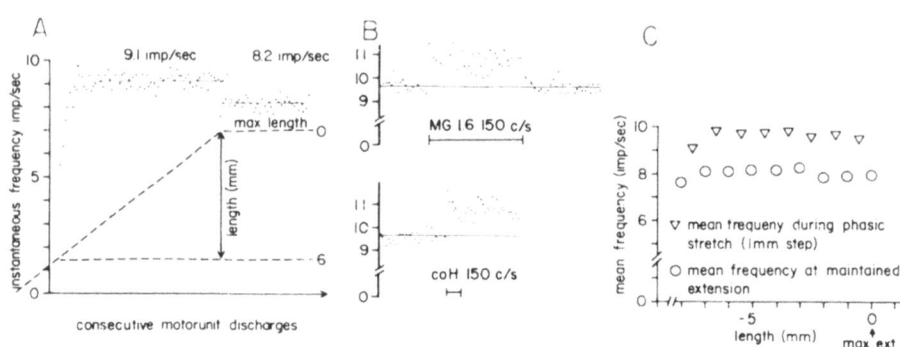

<u>Fig. 5</u>   The instantaneous discharge rate of motor units
              during slow constant muscle stretch, interrupted
              muscle stretch and during reflex activation
              superimposed on muscle stretch. A shows the dis-
              charge of a motor unit recorded with an electrode
              in the soleus muscle during slow extension of
              the muscle (0.8 mm/sec.). During the first few
              intervals after recruitment the discharge rate
              increases, but thereafter the level is quite
              constant throughout the extension, to decrease
              somewhat when holding the muscle at maximal ex-
              tension. B is a record from a motor unit dis-
              charging during maintained muscle stretch, when
              the nerve to the medial gastrocnemius is stimul-
              ated repetetively at a strength including the
              Ia fibers, giving heteronymous excitation. The
              rate is enhanced only during the period of
              stimulation whereas a similar stimulation of
              the nerve to the contralateral hamstring muscles
              gives an increase in the discharge rate which
              outlasts the stimulus (Grillner and Udo,unpubl.,
              Methods in 1971 a,b). C is recorded from another
              motor unit during intermittent extensions of
              1 mm at 0.8 mm/sec from recruitment of the motor
              unit to the max.extension. Note the remarkable
              constancy of the motor unit discharge rate at
              maintained extension at different levels of ex-
              tension, which indicates that no net excitation
              is added during 8 mm of muscle stretch. Note
              also the constancy of the dynamic response of
              the motor unit.

This is largely outside the range used in locomotion.
During lengthening at a constant low velocity, a fixed
number of motor units will be recruited at a short
muscle length, say around 90° in the ankle (Fig.4)
(Grillner and Udo,1971 b) and very few motor units will
be added thereafter (see Fig.7). The motor units will
after the initial recruitment remain at the same fre-

quency and no frequency modulation occurs throughout
the extension (Fig. 5 A,C) (Grillner and Udo,1971 a).
Thus in the steeper length range (Fig.7) a fixed number
of motor units will fire at a fixed frequency, i.e. any
change of tension in this range must be attributed to
the stiffness of the muscle.

Can the soleus muscle itself account for this stiffness? Motor units fire at maximal extension at a rate of
7.8±1.0 imp/sec. At this frequency it is apparent from
Fig. 2 and 6 A (nerve-muscle preparations) that the tension of the muscle will increase continuously up to the
maximal physiological extension, which has been determined with great accuracy (Grillner,1972). These data agree
rather well with the findings of Rack and Westbury (1969).
Note that these authors stretch the muscles several mm
beyond the maximal extension (30^0), which they also
write explicitely. The stiffness (increase in muscle
tension/mm extension) of the stretch reflex under good
conditions is between 90-100 g/mm, which can be compared
with the stiffness of the nerve-muscle preparation
stimulated at similar rates, which is 100-120 g/mm up to
a maximal extension. These two values agree and it
hence appears clearly that muscle stiffness is the chief
cause of the linear increase of tension in the steep
part of the stretch reflex up to maximal extension (Grillner and Udo,1971 a,b).

What happens if other inputs added to the stretch
reflex such as Ia-excitation from synergists or excitation from contralateral afferents (see Matthews,1959)?
Fig. 5 B,C shows that such repetitive stimulation increases the frequency of a motor unit tonically discharging due to muscle stretch (Grillner and Udo,1971
a and unpublished). Thus the muscle will follow a different length-tension curve, with stretch + nerve stimulation as compared with stretch alone. If the stiffness
of the muscle fibers is responsible for the slope of
the length-tension curve, this would mean that the stretch
reflex should not always during such combined stretch
and nerve stimulation increase monotonously up to the
maximal extension but rather reach a plateau due to the
shape of the length-tension curve (Fig. 6A). Precisely
this finding (Fig. 6B) was reported by Matthews (1959).
Hence the available evidence shows that stiffness of
the muscle fibers will be a very important factor
quantitatively; any study of the stretch reflex has to
consider this fact.

These results being crucial (Grillner,1970; Grillner and Udo,1971 a,b) for the interpretation P.B.C.

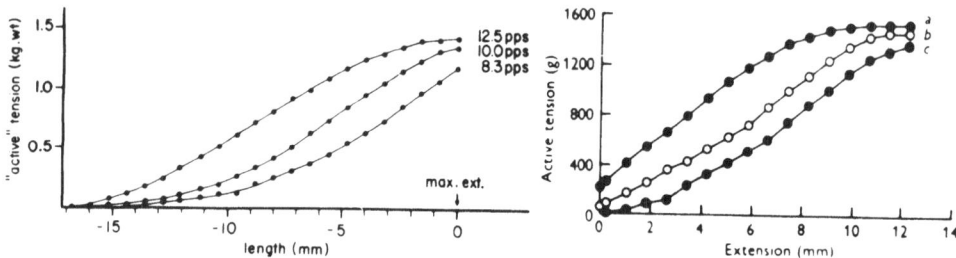

Fig. 6   Muscle stiffness of a soleus nerve-muscle pre-
          paration compared with the tonic stretch reflex
          during stretch with and without concomitant
          reflex stimulation. The left graph shows the
          length-tension diagram of a soleus muscle stimul-
          ated by means of distributed stimulation of five
          bundles of the ventral roots at the frequency
          indicated. The ordinate shows the active tension
          at different lengths which means that the tension
          contributed by passive factors has been subtract-
          ed from the total tension. For comparison the
          right graph shows Fig. 8 from Matthews (1959)
          in which c shows a normal soleus stretch reflex,
          whereas in the other curves the effect of
          electrical stimulation of the nerve to medial
          gastrocnemius at 90 c/s (a) and 55 c/s (b) is
          shown

Matthews (1969) has given, it seems appropriate to
comment once more on his suggestion that secondary endings contribute significantly to the tension in the
stretch reflex, since he has repeated his arguments unchanged recently (1972). The assumption used by Matthews
(1969, 1970) is that the length tension curve is flat
during the last 7 mm from max.extension, and therefore
the lack of occlusion between stretch and vibration must
be due to excitation from afferents not influenced by
vibration, such as the secondary endings. The present
results show that this basic assumption is incorrect
and that the muscle stiffness on the contrary is high
(Fig. 6A). This affects the interpretation of virtually
all his results as summarized below. The discharge rate
of a spindle afferent might be 25 imp/sec at -5 mm from
max.extension (see Eldred, Granit and Merton,1953) and
40 imp at max. extension. If at these two lengths a
vibration of 200 c/s is applied all spindle primaries
are assumed to be driven at this frequency . The vibration will add 175 imp/sec at   5 mm (cf. Fig. 7) and
160 imp/sec at max.extension. The difference between
175 and 160 is rather small and the excitation added

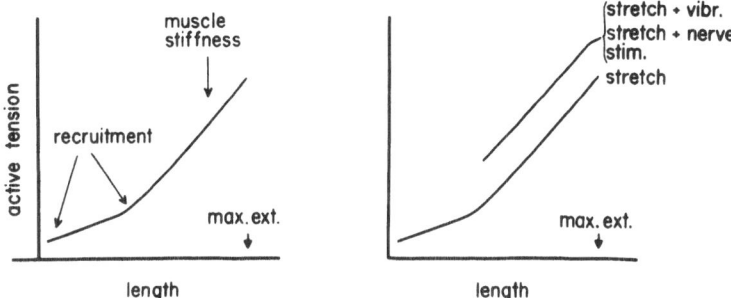

<u>Fig. 7</u>   Schematic representation of events during a
           tonic stretch reflex elicited by slow extension
           at constant velocity. The left graph is a
           schematic plot of active tension versus muscle
           length summarizing the results of Grillner and
           Udo (1971 a,b). The right graph shows typical
           findings in tonic stretch reflex activity with
           and without superimposition of a nerve stimula-
           tion or longitudinal vibration of the muscle

from the spindles should be approximately the same at
both max.extension and -5 mm. During vibration there
will be an increase of motor unit frequency (Brown,
Lawrence and Matthews, 1968; Grillner and Udo,unpublish-
ed). At each length which we choose to vibrate, we will
thus add approximately the same amount of excitation
leading to an increase in motor unit frequency and there-
by moving from one length-tension curve (Fig. 7 cf. Fig.
6 A) to another. As we stretch the muscle its stiffness
will add a large amount of tension in itself. If we
then vibrate at the new length we will again move from
one curve to another and expect approximately the same
increase in tension. These facts automatically invalid-
ate the arguments for the group II hypothesis used by
Matthews (1969) as illustrated in his table 1 and Figs.
1,2,3,4,5 and the discussion concerning occlusion. His
results can in fact be predicted if the muscle stiffness,
the motor unit frequency and the frequency modulation
from vibration or other extra inputs (see Fig. 7 of
this paper) is taken into consideration.

     Matthews, in his Figs. 6 and 7, makes a comparison
of the effect of stretch + vibration and stretch + nerve
stimulation (heteronymous Ia). He finds that independent
of the level of stretch, nerve stimulation and vibration
adds the same amount of tension (see Fig. 7 of this

paper). This is exactly what is to be   expected (cf.
above) and these findings can in no way be used to exclude that the muscle stiffness is of importance. His
results with small sudden stretch do not influence the
group II argument. However, another approach is used in
his Fig. 10 when recording the integrated electroneuro-
gram from a filament (3 expt) to lateral gastrocnemius
while vibrating the entire triceps surae at different
muscle lengths. He finds a larger response at maximal
length than at shorter muscle length. Since the primary
endings are assumed to be firing at the same rate while
vibrated independently of the length, these results
would indicate that excitation is added via some other
length-dependent mechanisms. This is the only argument
by Matthews (1969) that can be used to support the group
II hypothesis. But this experiment bears little weight
since the approach with vibration is built on the assumption that primary endings are selectively activated
in the amplitude and length range used. The evidence
for this is good for the soleus but is lacking for the
gastrocnemius. They are built in a different way and it
is quite uncertain how vibration affects the gastrocnemius (P.B.C. Matthews pers. comm.).

Another kind of indirect approach is used by Mc
Grath and Matthews (1970) when comparing the effect of
vibration before and after paralyzing small fibers in
the muscle nerve such as gr. II and III afferents and
γ - efferents. The effect of vibration is reduced after
procain, which would be expected if the gr. II afferents
were excitatory in the stretch reflex. On the other
hand, after procain block afferent activity from the
muscle in Ia, gr.II and III afferents is reduced tonically. This can well influence the "resting" excitability
of the α -motoneurones through spinal as well as supraspinal circuits regulating the long-term excitability
of α and γ -motoneurones via descending systems. The
situation is so much changed that it does not seem
meaningful to compare the effect of vibration before
and after procain.

The argument between Matthews and myself concerns
mainly whether the muscle stiffness is negligible for
the last 7 mm or large enough to account for the stiffness of the stretch reflex. Another quite independent
piece of evidence not discussed hitherto (see Grillner
and Udo,1971 a) is the discharge patterns of the motor
units. Fig. 5 in the paper shows that the motor unit
response while stretching intermittently at a rate of

0.8 mm/sec gives a quite considerable dynamic increase
in discharge rate, which is constant between different
levels of extension. Note also that the frequency varies
very little both at steady state and during stretch;
there is no reason to think that the motoneurones should
be saturated. Thus there is virtually no net excitatory
inflow added between different levels of maintained
stretch (last 8 mm) or dynamic stretch, i.e. the excitatory and inhibitory stretch evoked effects on the discharging motoneurones cancel each other. Matthews used
the last 7 mm and it follows from these results that in
discharging motor units no net excitation is added in
the length range at which the very strong gr. II excitation is assumed to act. The only ending that could give
the dynamic effect observed during each period of
stretch is the primary ending. Hence the excitation from
these endings seems to be quite potent, under stretch
reflex conditions.

After blockade of Ia afferents, group II afferents
give inhibition sometimes, however, quite negligible,
(Cangiano and Lutzemberger,1972; cf. Cook and Duncan,
1971). If repetitive stimulation of a synergist nerve
at a strength including group II afferents is superimposed on a stretch reflex this will result in inhibition of the stretch reflex (Matthews,1969). These data
indicate that there is no direct excitatory path from
secondary endings to motoneurones acting in the stretch
reflex. Under some conditions, however, electrically
stimulated group II afferents can provide some excitatory
effects. Westbury (1971) working on deeply anaesthetized
cats without tonic stretch reflexes, compared the effect
of stretch and vibration of the entire triceps surae
by recording motoneurones intracellularly. He concludes
in a short note that his results support Matthews' hypothesis. It should be cautioned again that vibration of
triceps surae is in no way proven to be a tool as selective as it is in soleus. One furhter piece of evidence
pertinent to this discussion is the finding that secondary endings can remove some presynaptic inhibition from
the terminals of Ia afferents (Pompeiano pers. comm.);
on the other hand, consider the results of Fig. 5 C in-
dicating that virtually no net excitation is added during the last 7 mm, when the group II excitation of Matthews is assumed to act.

On the whole, the available evidence indicates that
the primary endings give at least the main excitatory
effects in the tonic stretch reflex of the decerebrate
cat, whereas secondaries give virtually no effect or

inhibition. To understand the stretch reflex the muscle
properties must be taken into consideration.

Although an increased activity in secondaries does
not seem to increase the net excitation in the stretch
reflex, it will in all likelihood influence the excitation caused by muscle stretch, through the inhibitory
reflex path from group II afferents to motoneurones (a
possible function?). The resulting net excitation would
be the sum of the stretch evoked excitation and inhibition. The inhibitory pathway from group II afferents is
controlled from the brain stem. In all preparations in
which a stretch reflex is known to exist there is a depression of the transmission in this inhibitory pathway
to motoneurones (Grillner, 1969; Grillner and Udo,1970;
Ahlman, Grillner and Udo,1971).

It is inconceivable, that the main role of the
secondaries should be to provide generalized synaptic
effects of the flexor reflex type, rather we must admit
that our knowledge of the spinal control of movement is
still superficial and not despair for not yet having
found a meaningful role for the secondaries.

Force development during locomotion in relation to
muscle and reflex mechanisms
        The discussion above applies mostly to relatively
stable conditions as during standing. The situation
differs in locomotion. During the stance phase,i.e. the
period of the stepcycle when the foot is in contact
with the ground, the ankle angle decreases,i.e. the
muscle lengthens initially under the weight of the body
to subsequently shorten again (Fig. 8 A). In a fast gallop the time from touching the ground to the maximal
yield (the muscle then lengthens up to 15 mm at a speed
of 450 mm/sec) takes only 31 msec (Goslow et al.,1972).
Is this compatible with any kind of reflex regulation
of the force development in the yield, be it excitation
or inhibition? The answer is no. If a reflex input increases or decreases the frequency of already discharging motoneurones, there is a lag of between 20-30 msec
from the activation of ventral root fibers until any
change of tension occurs (see Grillner,1972). This value
will, however, be shorter if considering a twitch or
freshly recruited motor units; Melville-Jones and Watt
(1971) obtained, however, a value between 20-30 msec for
the electromechanical coupling in humans when observing
the resulting change in tension during asynchronous
natural activation of the muscle. To obtain the total
reflex time efferent, afferent and central delays must

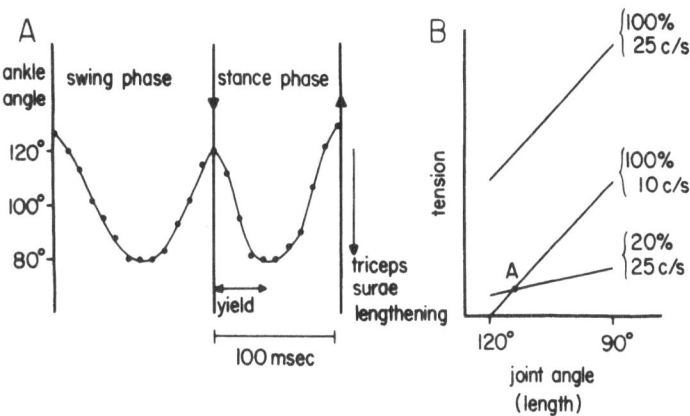

Fig. 8   Schematic representation of the ankle joint
          angles in gallop and comparison of the gain at
          high and low motor unit frequencies. The left
          graph is replotted from Engberg and Lundberg
          (1969) and indicates the joint angles in a slow
          gallop during the different phases of a loco-
          motor cycle. The right graph represents the gain
          (g/mm) in an imaginary ankle muscle during activ-
          ity at high and low frequency when 100% of the
          motor units are active and for comparison the
          gain if only 20% of the motor units are activated
          at high frequency which should give the same
          tension at the point A as the activity in the
          fully activated muscle at a lower frequency

be added as well as delays for receptor activation. The
shortest reflex time for the onset of change in tension
must be around 30 msec or more and very much longer until the tension has reached a steady level (Grillner,
1972). If the latency for the "functional stretch reflexes" should be included, at least another 20 msec
should be added (Hammond,1960; Melville-Jones and Watt,
1971). It follows in any case that a reflex induced when
the foot is put on the ground will influence the tension
only late in the stance phase (fast locomotion) and thus
a reflex control can simply not influence the same phase

of the movement, e.g. the tension in the yield cannot be influenced by events in the early stance phase. During slow movements, however, an effective reflex control can well occur but nevertheless it follows that the muscle contraction and the subsequent tension output in the first part of stance phase including the yield must be essentially determined prior to the stance phase itself and consequently the autoregulatory reflexes cannot be crucial for the movement programme, although it might assist and regulate during slower movements (Grillner, 1972; Melville-Jones and Watt, 1971).

Rather little is known about the force requirements during locomotion, but fortunately Manter (1938) measured the vertical and horizontal forces during the slow walk of the cat. From his data the net force developed by the ankle extensors has been calculated in Fig. 9 (for details see Grillner, 1972). The step cycle is in slow walk, and then the yield is smaller than during fast locomotion (Fig. 9 A). The force required during the stance phase increases to be maximal at the peak of the yield, when the length of the muscle is maximal and the limb carries the maximal load. It seems as if the muscles lengthen under the weight of the body which will by itself result in an increased muscle force (see Fig. 2) due to the length-tension curve of the muscle. Fig. 9 B shows the same data as A but plotted as force versus length. The relation between length and force is apparent although there appears to be a hysteresis phenomenon. A similar curve is obtained by sinusoidal stretch of a nerve-muscle preparation (Rack, 1966). In fact the force output and length changes in the stance phase might be explained by an activation of the muscles for a given period of time starting just prior to the stance phase and terminating in its later part. The resulting length changes being dependent on the load of the limb and the degree of activation of the extrafusal muscle which decides the resulting length. As the speed of locomotion increases, the yield increases and there are all reasons to believe that more force is required which could result partially from the lengthening of the muscle. The findings of Cavagna (Dusman and Margaria (1968) (also Bergel, Brown, Butler and Zacks, 1972) are very relevant for stepping. They find that a muscle will give rise to a larger force during shortening if the shortening is preceded by an active lengthening than if it starts from an isometric contraction; during locomotion a lengthening contraction always precedes the shortening.

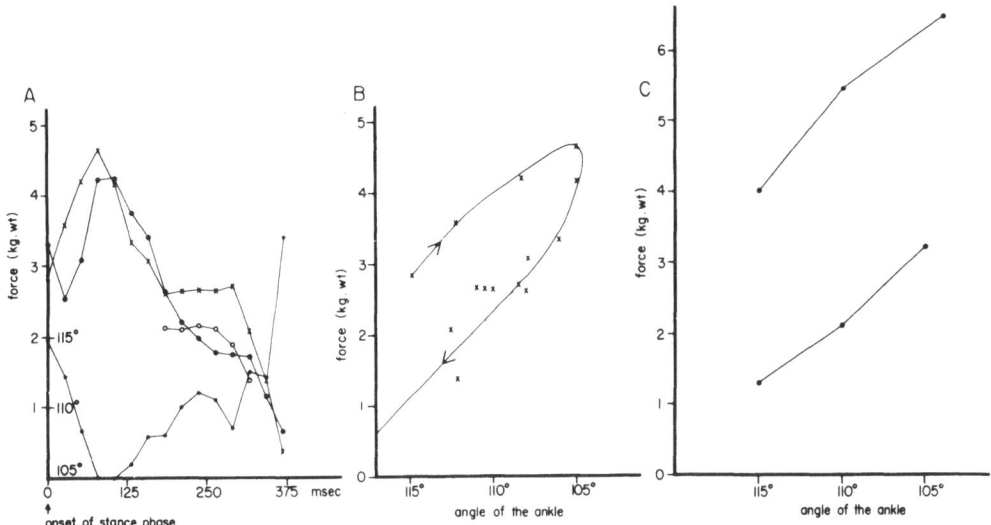

Fig. 9   Forces developed by the ankle extensors during
locomotion (slow walk). A shows the ankle joint
angles in slow walk as measured by Manter (1938)
and also the net forces that the ankle extensors
must develop in this same step cycle. The values
are obtained from a calculation of Manter's
measurements of vertical and horizontal forces.
B shows the same data as A but plotted as force
versus joint angle (length). C shows for comparison the stiffness of a lateral gastrocnemius
muscle in this length region

      From the beginning of the stance phase to the
maximum of the yield the force increases sharply to a
peak value, hence there seems to be no need for an inhibition of the motoneuronal activity during this period,
which has been postulated to be the function of the
Golgi tendon organs; moreover during fast locomotion
there is anyway no time for a reflex control of the
yield initiated in the stance phase. All muscle activity
must then be set in advance,i.e. being preprogrammed.
On this preset extrafusal activity the load will act to
finally result in a muscle length that changes with time
as does the load.

      Now if we return to the length-tension diagrams of
Fig. 2 it is clear that the curves for different frequencies of motor unit activity run in parallel although

they reach their maxima at different lengths. During
posture relatively low frequencies are used (for comparison see the tonic stretch reflex value of around
8 imp/sec), whereas during locomotion a quite different
range is used: 15-55 imp/sec (Shik,Orlovsky, Severin,
1966) with a rather constant rate for each motoneurone.
This means that length and tension will follow a curve
more to the left, in Fig. 2 the tension will be appreciable also at a short muscle length (120°) but it will
increase sharply throughout the range used in locomotion. The steepness for the different curves is obtained
with the same number of motor units. If the number of
motor units is reduced to 50%, the stiffness will decrease proportionally in all curves; on the other hand,
it is not likely that a single motor unit will show the
same type of length-tension graph as does the whole
muscle during asynchronous activity at the same mean
rate. Perhaps that graph would be more similar to the
ones obtained with synchronous stimulation to the whole
nerve, provided that the muscle is homogenous (cf.Rack
and Westbury,1969). Hence the stiffness at any rate
of motor unit activity is primarily dependent on the
number of active motor units (i.e. in the range in which
the curves are roughly parallel).

If we wish to reach the point A in the graph 8 B
two possibilities exist: either to activate a large
proportion of the motor units at a low rate say 10 pps
and then have a large stiffness, or to activate 20% of
the motor units at a high rate but consequently with a
muscle stiffness being only 20% of that in the previous
case. During posture rather low forces are required but
since low frequencies are used a proportionally larger
number of motor units can participate which will allow
a larger muscle stiffness. During locomotion, faster
rates are used since a high force must be developed
also at short muscle length but still the stiffness
will be large.

This work was supported by the Swedish Medical
Research Council (Project No. B-14X-3026) and by "Lars
Wallengrens donation".

REFERENCES

AHLMAN H., GRILLNER S. and UDO M. (1971). The effect of
    5HTP on the static fusimotor activity and the tonic
    stretch reflex of an extensor muscle. Brain Res. 27:
    393-396.

BERGEL D.H., BROWN M.C., BUTLER R.G. and ZACKS R.M.(1972)
    The effect of stretching a contracting muscle on its
    subsequent performance during shortening. J.Physiol.
    (Lond.). 225: 21-22 P.
BROWN M.C., ENGBERG I. and MATTHEWS P.B.C. (1967)·The
    relative sensitivity to vibration of muscle receptors
    of the cat. J.Physiol. (Lond.). 192: 773-800.
BROWN M.C., LAWRENCE D.G. and MATTHEWS P.B.C. (1968)
    Reflex inhibition by Ia afferent input of spontaneously
    discharging γ-motoneurones in the decerebrate cat.
    J.Physiol. (Lond.). 198: 5-7 P.
CANGIANO A. and LUTZEMBERGER L. (1972). The action of
    selectively activated group II muscle afferent fibers
    on extensor motoneurones. Brain Res. 41: 475-478.
CAVAGNA G.A., DUSMAN B. and MARGARIA R. (1968).
    Positive work done by a previously stretched muscle.
    J.appl.Physiol. 24: 21-32.
COOK W.A.Jr. and DUNCAN C.C.Jr. (1971).Contribution of
    group I afferents to the tonic stretch reflex of the
    decerebrate cat. Brain Res. 33: 509-513.
ELDRED E., GRANIT R. and MERTON P.A. (1953). Supraspinal
    control of the muscle spindles and its significance.
    J.Physiol. (Lond.). 122: 498-523.
EMONET-DENAND F., JAMI L., JOFFROY M. and LAPORTE Y.
    (1972). Absence de réflex myotatic après blockage de
    la conduction dans les fibres du group I. C.R.Acad.Sci.
    (Paris). 274D: 1542-1545.
ENGBERG I. and LUNDBERG A. (1969). An electromyographic
    analysis of muscular activity in the hindlimb of the
    cat during unrestrained locomotion. Acta physiol.scand.
    75: 614-630.
GAMBARIAN P.P., ORLOVSKI G.N., PROTOPOPOVA T.Y., SEVERIN
    F.V. and SHIK M.L. (1971). The activity of muscles
    during different gaits and adaptive changes of moving
    organs in family Felidae. Morphology and ecology of
    vertebrates. Proc.Inst.Zool.Acad.Sci. USSR. 48: 220-239.
GOSLOW G.E.Jr., REINKING R.M. and STUART D.G. (1972).
    The cat step cycle: hindlimb joint angles and muscle
    lengths during unrestrained locomotion. J.Morphology
    (in press).
GRANIT R. (1970). The Basis of Motor Control. Academic
    Press,London and New York.
GRILLNER S. (1969). The influence of DOPA on the static
    and the dynamic fusimotor activity to the triceps
    surae of the spinal cat. Acta physiol.scand. 77: 490-
    509.
GRILLNER S. (1970). Is the tonic stretch reflex depend-
    ent upon group II excitation? Acta physiol.scand. 78:
    431-432.

GRILLNER S. (1972). The role of muscle stiffness in
    meeting the changing postural and locomotor require-
    ments for force development by the ankle extensors.
    Acta physiol.scand. (in press).
GRILLNER S. and UDO M. (1970). Is the tonic stretch
    reflex dependent on suppression of autogenetic in-
    hibitory reflexes? Acta physiol scand. 79: 13-14 A.
GRILLNER S. and UDO M. (1971ᵃ). Motor unit activity and
    stiffness of the contracting muscle fibres in the
    tonic stretch reflex. Acta physiol.scand. 81: 422-424.
GRILLNER S. and UDO M. (1971ᵇ). Recruitment in the tonic
    stretch reflex. Acta physiol.scand. 81: 571-573.
HAMMOND P.H. (1960). An experimental study of servoaction
    in human muscular control. Proc.Third Intern.Conf.Med.
    Electr. (London). Part 2: 190-199.
LAPORTE Y. and BESSOU P. (1959). Modifications d'excita-
    bilité de motoneurones homonymes provoquées par l'ac-
    tivation physiologique de fibres afférentes d'origine
    musculaire du group II. J.Physiol. (Paris). 51: 897-908.
MANTER J.T. (1938). The dynamics of quadrupedal walking.
    J.exp.Biol. 15: 522-540.
MATTHEWS P.B.C. (1959). A study of certain factors in-
    fluencing the stretch reflex of the decerebrate cat.
    J.Physiol. (Lond). 147: 547-564.
MATTHEWS P.B.C. (1969). Evidence that the secondary as
    well as the primary endings of the muscle spindles
    may be responsible for the tonic stretch reflex of the
    decerebrate cat. J.Physiol. (Lond.).204: 365-393.
MATTHEWS P.B.C. (1970). A reply to criticism of the
    hypothesis that the group II afferents contribute ex-
    citation to the stretch reflex. Acta physiol.scand.
    79: 431-433.
MATTHEWS P.B.C. (1972). Mammalian muscle receptors and
    their central actions. London, Edward Arnold (Publi-
    shers) Ltd.
McGRATH G.Y. and MATTHEWS P.B.C. (1970). Support for an
    autogenetic excitatory reflex action of the spindle
    secondaries from the effect of gamma blocade by pro
    caine. J.Physiol. (Lond.). 210: 176-177 p.
MELVILLE JONES G. and WATT D.G.D. (1971). Observations
    on the control of stepping and hopping movements in
    man. J.Physiol. (Lond.). 219: 709-727.
RACK P.M.H. (1966). The behaviour of a mammalian muscle
    during sinusoidal stretching. J.Physiol.(Lond.). 183:
    1-14.
RACK P.M.H. (1970). The significance of mechanical pro-
    perties of muscle in the reflex control of posture,
    pp. 317-322. In Excitatory Synaptic Mechanisms. Oslo.
    Universitetsforlaget.

RACK P.M.H. and WESTBURY D.R. (1969). The effects of
    length and stimulus rate on tension in the isometric
    cat soleus muscle. J.Physiol.(Lond.) 204: 443-460.
SEVERIN F.V., SHIK M.L. and ORLOVSKI G.N. (1967). Work
    of muscles and single motoneurones during controlled
    locomotion. Biofizika. (eng.translation). 12: 762-772.
SHICK M.L., DILOVSKY G.N., SEVERIN F.V. (1966). Organiza-
    tion of locomotive synergy. Biofizika (in Russian).
    11: 879-887.
TAUB E. and BERMAN A.J. (1968). Movement and learning
    in the absence of sensory feedback, pp.173-192. In:
    The Neurophysiology of Spatially Oriented Behaviour.
    Ed. S.J.Freedman. The Dorsey Press, Homewood, Illinois,
    Irwing-Dorsey Ltd., Nobleton, Ontario.
WESTBURY D.R. (1971). A comparison of stretch and vibra-
    tion reflexes at the motoneurone. J.Physiol. (Lond.)
    213: 25-26
WETZEL M.C., GERLACH R.L., STERN L.Z. and HANNAPEL L.K.
    (1972). Behaviour and histochemistry of functionally
    isolated cat ankle extensors. Experimental Neurology.
    (in press).

THE CONTROL OF POSTURE AND LOCOMOTION

V. S. Gurfinkel and M. L. Shik

From the Institute of the Problems of
Information Transmission
Moscow, USSR

In this paper we have attempted to concentrate not
so much on the apparent differences between standing
and walking but rather on the common mechanisms shared
by both actions. The analysis of the natural movements
shows that during these two actions there is not only
a successive change of postural and motor stabilisation
modes but also a simultaneous realization of these two
modes. In a multicomponent system with an elaborate
communication network such as the vertebrate locomotor
apparatus, the movement of some components provoke a
corresponding reaction in other components. When precise
movements are produced there arises the necessity to
prevent the reactive movements of distant components
by stabilizing their position. This postural activity
is carried out simultaneously with the macromovements.

It should be noted that the changes in postural
activity have not only a compensating, but also an anticipatory character. Usually they precede the macromovements and take into account the expected result of the
movement (Belenkiy, Gurfinkel and Paltsev,1967).

This simultaneously functioning mechanism of postural and motor control is particularly important for
the dynamic stabilization of the body during locomotion.

While most students of locomotor behaviour believe
that locomotion is organized according to a central
program continuously readjusted by the inflow of peri-
pheric information, this view is not generally shared

by the workers interested in postural control, who seem
to underestimate the role of the central program and to
concentrate mainly on the different aspects of afferent
information.

Such approach to the problem would be valid in a
model investigation of the stabilization of a two-com-
ponent system, but in more complex types of postural
activity, such as maintaining of the vertical posture,
underestimation of the central program is indefendable.
Here is an example. Many investigators have shown that
postural stabilization is a dynamic process, characterized by continuous oscillations of the center of gravity. These oscillations are random and, in a two-compon-
ent system are known as tremor of active posture.

However in a multi-element system this background
is affected by periodic disturbances due to circulation
and respiration.

If the stretch-reflex, gamma-system (Merton,1953)
and the role of the delay in this reflex (Marschall
and Walsh,1956; Lippold,1970) are sufficient to explain
the mechanism of the active posture stabilization, a
model working according to a definite program is necessary in order to explain the mechanisms of compensation
of the spinal column respiratory movements and internal
organ displacements (respiratory synergy of the vertical
posture (Gurfinkel, Kotz, Paltsev and Feldman,1971).

Nonetheless the majority of investigations devoted
to the analysis of postural activity has for objective
to find out the role of various reflexes involved in
posture stabilization.

For several decades it has become widely accepted
that three main sensor modalities participate in the
regulation of the vertical posture: proprioception,
vision and vestibular apparatus. Recent investigations,
carried out in man give additional data on the importance of these afferent systems for postural control.

1. THE ROLE OF THE STRETCH-REFLEX IN
THE CONTROL OF POSTURE

The stretch-reflex holds a key-position in all the
theories of the mechanism of postural regulation.

The impulses coming from the muscle receptors are essential for maintaining a certain level of motoneurone activity. The stretch-reflex can, however, be used for a more special postural task, namely to provide a finer control of rapid equilibrium reactions.

That is why much attention has been accorded to study of the stretch-reflex system in active posture.

It is known that when the Subject is at rest, only a phasic stretch-reflex can be evoked. It requires considerable change in the length of the muscle and great velocity of extention.

In the process of stabilization of the equilibrium the changes in the length of the muscle amount to 0.1 mm and are executed at a speed of 0.1 mm/sec.

Obviously, in order to be effective as a stabilizing mechanism, the stretch-reflex should have a different order of sensitivity during postural activity and at rest.

In the work of Agarwal Berman and Stark,(1970) Agarwal, Berman, Löhnberg and Stark,(1970) the properties of the stretch-reflex involved in the stabilization of the posture have been studied and simulated.

Using the Achilles reflex as an example, the authors investigated different characteristics of the stretch-reflex and concluded that the system is non-linear. Investigations were carried out in recumbent Subjects. It was naturally supposed that in an erect posture many of the characteristics of the reflex/such as threshold, gain etc./ would change.

In our laboratory it was shown(Elner, Popov and Gurfinkel,1972) that the sensitivity of the stretch-reflex increased when passing from a sitting to an upright position. Thus the threshold of the electrical response of m.triceps surae to a stretch, performed by a 10^{0} dorsiflexion of the foot, is 40^{0}-50^{0} per sec. at rest. In vertical position it is twice as low and amounts to 20^{0}-30^{0} per sec. If the stretching of m.triceps surae takes place under a menace of falling(shift of the mobile horizontal platform) the stretch reaction threshold is 5^{0} per sec., that is it decreases 8 to 10 times. Simultaneously a considerable increase of the gain of the stretch-reflex is observed. But despite

such a decrease the threshold appears to be much higher
than the threshold required to perform the quick equilibrium reactions.

What is particular about our experiments is that
the value of the muscle elongation was rather large.
The sensitivity of m.gastrocnemius stretch-reflex of
the cat (Matthews, 1969) during small elongations (up
to 0.3 mm) is 2 to 4 times higher than during larger
elongations. This nonlinearity may be explained by the
greater sensitivity of the spindles at the beginning of
stretching (Brown, Goodwin and Matthews, 1969). These
authors assumed that this effect was due to the presence of closed actomyosin bridges in the intrafusal
fibers.

Of great interest are the data presented by Nashner
(1970), who studied the m.triceps surae reaction to a
gradual change of the ankle joint angle. He measured
the value of the reaction and calculated the value of
the joint moment. His measurements prove that the
stretch-reflex gain is a nonlinear function of the
stretch. Thus when due to the stretch of the ankle joint,
the foot is rotated in the ankle at an angle of 0.1°, the
gain of the stretch is twice as large as that at 0.25°
and 0.5° stretch.

To calculate the moment the author registered the
support reactions and the joint displacements. The value
of the support reactions was determined not only by a
true stretch response, but also by the so called pseudo-
stretch that depends upon the visco-elastic properties
of the muscle stretched.

During small changes of the length of the muscle
the resistance to stretch is higher than during greater
ones (Hill, D., 1968). The calculation of the active
part of the stretch reflex showed that the gain in
upright position accounts for only 1/3 of the effort
necessary to stabilize the body.

It should be noted that the decrease of the sensitivity of the stretch-reflex system by means of block-
ing the gamma-efferents does not particularly influence
the control of vertical posture (Shambes, 1969).

No noticeable deterioration of stability is observed during a prolonged occlusion of a.femoralis (up to
30 min.) although the Achilles reflex disappears (Mama-
sakhlisow, Elner and Gurfinkel, 1972). The required
level of motoneurone activity is presumably supported

by central structures responsible for the vertical
posture program. A decrease of muscle force (induced by
application of myorelaxant) decreases abruptly the stability, as it leads to slow oscillations of high amplitude.

2. THE ROLE OF THE VISUAL SYSTEM IN
VERTICAL POSTURE CONTROL

In a great number of works it has been shown that
a block of the visual input leads to equilibrium disturbances. Recent investigation has supplied new data
on this problem. Baron (1951) has proved that the extra-
ocular muscles exert considerable influence on the position of the body. For instance he showed that the position of the centre of gravity projection is displaced
in patients with strabismus and that a correction of
strabismus with prisms brings the centre of gravity to
the normal position. In healthy erect Subjects the position of the centre of gravity changes when the gaze is
shifted (Gantchev, Draganova and Dunev, 1972).

Previously it has been shown (Gurfinkel, Kots and
Shik, 1965; Gurfinkel and Elner, 1971) that the non-
visual function of the eye plays a definite role in
maintaining the vertical posture. The diffuse light
probably exerts an influence on the equilibrium mechanisms through the retino-teclal pathways. The vestibular
effects on the posture (galvanic probe) also depend on
the vision. Closing of the eyes facilitates the vestibular influences as well as disturbances of gaze fixation
(with normal illumination) and darkness (with unchanged
fixation). Fixation is of greater importance for stabilization than illumination (Njiokiktjien, 1972).

The ancient belief that postural stabilization and
locomotion are performed by different muscle groups is
gone into oblivion but another misconception is still
tenacious. The postural activity is supposed to be based on the system of stabilizing reflexes and primarily
on the stretch reflexes whereas the regulation of other
types of movements would be mostly achieved by a central program.

We believe that the natural types of postural
activity such as maintenance of the vertical position
are based on definite central programs and that is the
reason of our stressing the importance of the general
neural mechanisms, which underly the postural and other

types of motor activity.

   A program, that had been previously called the
scheme of the body can be mentioned here as an example.
A leading part in this program and its relations with
the environment belongs to the visual and the oculo-
motor apparatus. This program is realized not only
through the play of the thresholds and gain of reflexes
but also by directional shifts of reflex streams in accordance with the particular postural task (address
change). Lately some neurophysiological pathways through
which such an address change of reflexes could take place
have been suggested (by Hongo, Jankowska and Lundberg,
1969).

3. LOCOMOTION

   In postural activity the main control task is to
stabilize either the muscle force or the joint angle or
the position of the centre of gravity. If the fluctua-
tions of external forces, small and random factors such
as duration of the single contraction of muscle fibers
or the time circulation of the signal in the proprioceptive loop are responsible for microcyclic phenomena.
Tremor of such origin limits the accuracy of postural
stabilization.

   However in many movements - locomotion in particular - macrocyclicity is the essential feature, and the
duration of a cycle is determined by quite different
factors. Let us consider some typical properties of
quadrupedal locomotion (dog, cat). The step of the limb
is subdivided into swing and stance phases. In the swing
phase there is flexion in all three main joints followed by extension in the knee and ankle (elbow and wrist)
joints. In the stance phase the hip (shoulder) joint
extends and distal joints yield and then extend.

   When the velocity of locomotion changes, the durations of the different parts of a cycle change too, but
the basic pattern of the stepping limb - that is the
order of direction changes of movements in the three
main joints - persists. If one knows the movements in
one joint, it is possible to reconstruct the curves for
the other joints of the limb. This means that there is
an unity of action of a limb during locomotion.

   The nervous system can change the force exerted by
some muscles without disturbing the stepping pattern of

the limb. However, it is impossible to change radically
the order in which the muscles of a limb are activated,
because no stepping would result.

Only a few muscles can change substantially the'
type of their activity when the velocity of locomotion
changes (Engberg and Lundberg, 1969; Gambarian, Orlovsky, Protopopova, Severin and Shik, 1971). A few muscles
contract twice per cycle, but most of them generate
only one burst. Conventionally it is possible to divide
the muscles of a limb into two main groups, flexors and
extensors. But such a classification is not very accurate. First, it is not easy to relate the biarticular
muscles to a definite group according to their cinematic effect. Second, the timing of muscle activity during
a locomotor cycle is hard to describe in terms of such
a classification. The description according to which all
muscles of a limb are related to one of the two groups
alternately active is erroneous.Actually, certain
muscles are active at every moment of the cycle, but
the number of muscles simultaneously active has two
peaks: at the beginning of the swing phase and in the
middle of the stance phase (Gambarian et al., 1971).
However the phases of maximal activity do not coincide
in different muscles.

The movements of symmetrical hind (fore) limbs are
more loosely correlated than the movements at the different joints of one and the same limb. The hind limbs
are moved with half a cycle phase lag in walk and trot
and synphasically in gallop. In artificial conditions
one can observe even inequal durations of the cycles of
each hind limb during locomotion (Kulagin and Shik,
1970).

The correlation between the movements of the anterior and posterior limbs is still weaker. There are
no invariants of the locomotion velocity in fore-hind
limb relations. When the velocity of the diagonal locomotion of a dog changes from 2-3 to 7-8 km/h the phase
lag between the movements of diagonal fore- and hind
limbs decreases continuously from a quarter of a cycle
to zero. In that range of velocities the duration of
the stance phase diminishes almost three-fold, although the swing phase shortens less than 10%. Similarly, the changes in the velocity of the treadmill belt
during the induced locomotion in the mesencephalic cat
are followed by changes in the duration of the stance
phase, while the swing phase shortens insignificantly

(Shik, Severin and Orlovsky, 1966).

4. THE SPINAL AUTOMATISM OF THE STEPPING LIMB

Cinematic and electromyographic evidence suggest
that there exists an automatism of the stepping limb
which is responsible for a certain sequence of activity
of the muscles in a cycle and which can adapt the duration of the stance phase (correspondingly - the duration of activity of the main extensors) to the actual
velocity of locomotion, which depends not only on the
activity of the animal, but on the properties of the
road and other factors (Orlovsky, Severin and Shik,
1966). Neurophysiological data prove that such an automatic mechanism exists in the spinal cord. A century
ago Holtz and Freusberg observed stepping of hind limbs
in a chronic spinal dog suspended in vertical position.
In the decapitated cat Roaf and Sherrington (1910)
elicited stepping of a hind limb by high-frequency
stimulation of a certain point on the section of the
cord at the C_1 level. It is possible to evoke the stepping of hind limbs in an acute spinal cat by nociceptive
stimulation of peri-anal region (Sherrington, 1910) or
after intravenous injection of di-hydroxy-phenilalanin
(DOPA) (Grillner, 1969; Budakova, 1971). Even in a
curarized spinal animal under Nialamid and DOPA it is
possible to observe sometimes an alternating activity
in nerves of antagonist muscles of a hind limb (Jankowska, Jukes, Lund and Lundberg, 1967a, b; Viala and Buser,
1971).

Thus the spinal cord is capable to generate stepping at least of the hind limbs, but this automatic
mechanism in the acute isolated cord must be activated
or released. Although there is no doubt about the exist-
ance of such an automatism there are only hypotheses
about its structure. One of the first hypotheses (Philipson, 1905) considered stepping as a chain-reflex. It
is true that cyclic afferent input is very essential
(Gray, 1950), but stepping is not a chain-reflex. Deafferented hind limbs of the dog and the monkey (Taub and
Berman, 1968) with intact brain and of the acute mesencephalic cat take part in locomotion (in the last
case - during induced locomotion on treadmill). But
when the fore limbs of the mesencephalic cat are held,
the hind limbs cease their activity immediately or,
more rarely, in the next 1-3 cycles, although the
stimulation of the midbrain "locomotor region" continues
(Shik, Orlovsky and Severin, 1966). This means that the

cyclic afferent input from the intact fore limbs, which
bears no information about muscles and joints of hindlimbs, is sufficient to induce stepping movements of
the hind limbs. A change of duration of the forelimb
cycle, due to changing the speed of the treadmill belt,
is followed by a corresponding change of duration of
the deafferented hindlimb cycle.

Thus the activity of the intraspinal programm of
stepping is dependent essentially on the afferent and
descending flow, but it cannot be considered only as a
mechanism for classifying of specific receptor inflow
as assumed by the chain - reflex hypothesis. The idea
about the structure of the intraspinal program of
stepping was originally proposed by Brown (1914). He
supposed that the "half - centers" of the antagonist
muscles of a limb were linked by mutually inhibitory,
reciprocal, connections. When one of the "half-centers"
is active, the other would be inhibited. During its
activity the "half-center" becomes "tired" continuously,
its inhibitory influence on the antagonistic "half-
center" is diminishing. At some time the activity of
the antagonist "half-center" prevails, then the first one
is inhibited, and activity of the second one increases
rapidly up to a maximum. The process has a cyclic course
even when the input to this system is tonic.

The basic idea of Brown can often be found in
modern work. The most important progress has been realized by Jankowska et al., 1967a, b Lundberg, 1969   They
demonstrated that the reciprocal inhibition is achieved
through inhibitory interneurones. These interneurones
are usually silent in the spinal cat but they can be
activated by DOPA injection (Jankowska et al., 1967a, b).
Lundberg assumes that the same group of interneurones
activate both the motoneurones of a given pool and inhibitory interneurones which project to the excitatory
interneurones in the antagonistic pool. Lundberg suggests
also that the specific proprioceptive reflexes are responsible for the activation of some muscles out of phase
with one of two main groups. A third modification of the
"half-center" hypothesis is discussed by mathematicians.
They claim that by postulating the existence of interneuronal subpopulations with different thresholds we
substitute the ill-founded supposition that neurones
become "tired" during their activity (J.Feldman, 1972).

The hypothesis of reciprocal "half-centers" deals
with the problem of alternative activity of the antagonists, but this is only a part of the problem of the

general temporal organization of the activity of the
muscles of the stepping limb. This hypothesis does not
consider the adaptation of the duration of the cycle
to the rate of locomotion, in particular the dispropor-
tional changes in the duration of stance and swing
phases. Reciprocal interaction of "half-centers" is
rather a universal mechanism always involved in the
alternating activity of antagonists, but in the different
types of movements, as in stepping and scratching, it
must be supplemented by various, more specialized
programs.

Another hypothesis was introduced recently by
Szekely and Czeh (1971). Observing the twitches in different forelimb muscles during microstimulation of the
cervical spinal cord in Urodela and recording the EMG
of the forelimb muscles in these animals during locomotion, these investigators were led to elaborate the
hypothesis of "microcycles":

"... it seems as if the motor column could be divided
into neuronal assemblies of arbitrary extent, which
represent a set of muscles, each in different combination. Groups of motor neurones representing individual
muscles within these assemblies are interconnected by
excitatory and inhibitory interneurones in such a manner that they are firing consecutively, giving rise to
a cyclic activity. The assemblies are, furthermore, so
intercoupled that the many small cycles they generate
fit together and result in the single large cycle of
the walking step".

The coordination of a great number of such gener-
ators and their adaptation to the rate of locomotion
is certainly a difficult task. A further complication
arises from the enormous number of interneurones necessary to build up a large number of individual cycles
with periods of the order of seconds. This problem is
particularly striking in the spinal cord of amphibia
given its very modest total interneuronal population
(Nieuwenhuys, 1964).

It is interesting to note that, undoubtedly, the
swimming of the fishes is due to the propagation of
some type of activity along the body axis, which in-
volves consecutively the muscles of the different
somites. The reciprocal mechanism responsible for the
alternating activity of the symmetrical muscles of the
somite is of course essential for swimming, but nobody

maintains that it could be substituted to the activity
propagated along the body axis.

Of course, it is hard to imagine such a "fishy"
mechanism governing the pedestral locomotion. Nevertheless we believe that some features of this mechanism
are retained in the control of stepping limb. We believe
that a circular trajectory ("ring") is established in
such a way that all the motoneurones of the muscles of
a limb are activated in an appropriate pattern. This
"ring" is not a linear chain of interneurones. At each
cross-section of time it has a certain number of active
neurones, a function of the afferent and efferent inflow. The change of pattern depends on the interaction
of spatial and temporal summation. Thus the local velocity of propagation of activity along the "ring" can
be different in its different segments. The stance
part of the ring is especially succeptible to afferent
input. The duration of different parts of the cycle can
be controlled more or less independently. Since the
synaptic delay cannot be shorter than a certain value
and the minimal velocity of propagation of activity
along the ring is limited by the summation time, the
range of duration of the stepping cycles would be subjected to these constraints. If, in the absence of afferent input the speed of propagation of the activity
in some segments of the ring falls to a near-threshold
value, the possibility of disruption of the cycle would
become appreciable. From this point of view it is clear,
why several start cycles are necessary until a stability
of stepping is achieved in induced locomotion in the
mesencephalic cat.

In the mesencephalic cat the duration of stance
phase and the mean amplitude of the electromyogram of
the main muscles of the limb seem to be controlled independently. The first is dependent on the velocity of
the treadmill belt, the second, on the strength of
activation of the midbrain locomotor centres. A certain
amount of inhibitory interneurones would be required
to achieve that aim as well as to provide an unidirec-
tional propagation of the activity along the ring and
to control the length of the active segment of the ring.

The ring hypothesis is not inconsistent with the
half-centre theory. On the one hand the ring circuit
can be complemented by the reciprocal interaction of
antagonists; on the other the reciprocal relations can
be viewed as a particular case of the ring circuit.

This would be the case when the rate of propagation of
the activity during the larger part of the stance and
the swing phases is extremely low in respect to the
velocity in the transition segments. In this case both
proposed circuits would be equivalent. Alhough there is
no direct experimental evidence for the ring hypothesis
it could explain a large number of experimental data.

The most probably interneurone set which could
realize such a ring is the non-specific neurone.pool
which forms a column in the dorsolateral part of the
ventral horn (Westman and Bowsher, 1971). Jankowska
et al.(1967a, b) have shown that these neurones are
activated by DOPA and that they are responsible for the
reciprocal activity of motoneurones.

Under the influence of this drug, and after a
brief volley is applied to elicit the flexor reflex
these interneurones provoke, with a latency of 100 ms,
a long lasting (hundreds of ms) asynchronous activity
in the motoneurones which is most likely to be the car-
rier of the intraspinal stepping program. Thus Ludberg
and colleagues discovered a neuronal system in the
spinal cord, very different from oligosynaptic pathways.

Morphological investigation (Scheibel and Scheibel,
1966; Sterling and Knypers, 1968) has shown that many
if not most of the ventral horn interneurones are in
fact "propriospinal neurones", that is they send their
axons in the neighbouring segments too. For Ia inhibitory interneurones this is now proved also electro-
physiologically by Jankowska and Roberts (1972). Strictly speaking this fact is indifferent to the different
hypotheses concerning the organization of stepping
program. However, it is to be noted that the "ring"
hypothesis is essentially multisegmental while the
reciprocal mechanism can be considered as rather intra-
segmental.

The interlimb coordination can be achieved by the
interaction of different loops through the propriospinal (Barilari and Knypers, 1969; Miller, 1970),
spino-bulbo-spinal (Shimamura and Livingston, 1963) and
other systems, in particular those which involve the
cerebellum.

5. DUAL SIGNIFICANCE OF DESCENDING INFLUENCES

Since Roaf-Sherrington's experiment we know that
for the activation (release) of the spinal stepping
automatism a tonic descending input is sufficient. The
same conclusion can be drawn from the observation that
after DOPA-injection, a stepping of the hind limbs of
the spinal cat can be elicited. The changes in the state
of the spinal cord provoked by stimulation of the midbrain "locomotor region" in the mesencephalic cat are
similar to those, which were found originally by Jankowska et.al. (1967a, b) in the spinal cat after DOPA-
injection (Grillner and Shik, 1972). Therefore it is
probable, that the descending influences responsible
for the activation (release) of the spinal stepping
program are mediated by descending monoaminergic fibers,
as proposed orginally by Jankowska et al. (1967a, b).
This tonic inflow is the basic efferent influence in
locomotion.

However, during locomotion the large reticulo-,
vestibulo- and rubrospinal neurones generate spikes
with a frequency modulated in the locomotor rhythm
(Orlovsky, 1970; Orlovsky and Pavlova, 1972). This
modulation is due to ascending inflow. These myelinated
systems could influence primarily not the automatic
spinal stepping mechanism, but motoneurones and interneurones belonging to oligosynaptic reflex arcs. They
could be important also for the maintainance of equilibrium during locomotion. For space orientation the
corticofugal system may also be of importance. Thus it
seems reasonable to consider the descending influence
during locomotion as consisting of two separate parts:
a basic inflow, responsible for the activation or release of the automatic spinal stepping program, and
the properly coordination circuit aimed at the motoneurones and interneurones of the oligosynaptic reflex
arcs.

6. BRAIN CONTROL OF LOCOMOTION

The acute mesencephalic cat cannot walk (Hinsey,
Ranson and McNattin, 1930), but the subthalamic one can.
Under light anaesthesia the stimulation of the sub-
thalamus can elicit running movements of the limbs
(Waller, 1940; Grossman, 1958). For a time it was be-
lieved that the subthalamus is a necessary structure of

the locomotion control system. However, Bard and Macht
(1958) and later Woods (1964) have shown that the
chronic mesencephalic cat and rat can walk. In the acute
mesencephalic cat locomotion can be induced by stimulation of the nucleus cuneiformis mesencephali (Horsley-
Clarke coordinates P2, L4, H0) (Shik et al., 1966;
Shik, 1971). In the chronic cat with destruction of the
centrum medianum-nucl. parafascicularis area, stimulation of the same midbrain "locomotor" region elicites
locomotion (Sirota and Shik, 1972). However, after a
lesion in the nucl. cuneiformis region, walking in the
otherwise intact cat is possible. Tower (1936) observed
running movements of the limbs lightly anaesthetized
pyramidotomized cat after stimulation of certain cortical fields (Shik, Orlovsky, Severin, 1968).

    Thus the locomotion control system includes the
spinal stepping automatism and two lower-brain stem
mechanisms: one activating (releasing) and the other
coordinating. These lower-brain stem mechanisms are
controlled by the cerebellum, midbrain "locomotor" region, subthalamus and cerebral cortex. The cerebellum is
essential for the interlimb coordination and equilibrium
maintenance. The midbrain "locomotor" region and subthalamus can release and activate the spinal automatism
of stepping through the lower brain stem. The subthalamus is important in the initiation of motivationally
conditioned locomotion. The cortical level is responsible at least for space orientation during locomotion.
Of course this hypothetical structuration needs to be
further investigated and verified.

                    R E F E R E N C E S

AGARWAL G.C., BERMAN B.M. and STARK L. (1970). Studies
    in postural control system. Part I. Torque disturb-
    ance input. IEEE Trans.on system science and cy-
    bernetics, v.SSC-6, 2, 116-121.
AGARWAL G.C., BERMAN B.M., L HNBERG P. and STARK L.(1970).
    Studies in postural control systems. Part. II. Tendon
    Jerk Input. IEEE Trans. on system science and cybern-
    etics, v.SSC-6, 2, 122-126.
BARD P. and MACHT M.B. (1958). The behaviour of chron-
    ically decerebrate cats. In Neurological basis of
    behaviour, ed. G.E.W. Wolstenholme and C.M.O. O'Con-
    nor, Ciba Found. Symp. pp. 55-71. London: Churchill.
BARILARI M.G. and KNYPERS G.J.M. (1969). Propriospinal
    fibers interconnecting the spinal enlargements in the
    cat, Brain Res. 14: 321-330.

BARON J.-B. (1951). Relation entre les muscles moteurs
    oculaires, les nageoires et l'equilibre des poissons.-
    C.R.Acad.Sc., 231: 1087-1088.
BELENKIY V.E., GURFINKEL V.S. and PALTSEV R.I. (1967).
    On the elements of voluntary movement control. Bio-
    fizika, 12: 135-141 (in Russian).
BROWN M.C., GOODWIN G.M. and MATTHEWS P.B.C. (1969).
    After effects of fusimotor stimulation on the response
    of muscle spindle primary afferent endings. J.Physiol.
    (Lond.) 205: 677-694.
BROWN T.G. (1914). On the nature of the fundamental
    activity of the nervous centres: together with an
    analysis of the rhythmic activity in progression and
    a theory of evolution of the function in the nervous
    system. J.Physiol.(Lond.) 48: 18-46.
BUDAKOWA N.N. (1971). Stepping movements evoked by a
    rhythmic stimulation of a dorsal root in mesencephalic
    cat. Sechenov Physiol. J. USSR, 57: 1632-1640 (in
    Russian).
ELNER A.M., POPOV K.E. and GURFINKEL V.S. (1972). Chang-
    es of the stretch reflex state during the muscle act-
    ivity in man. In Abstr. Sec.Intern.Symp.Motor Control,
    Varna 1972, p.50 (in Russian).
ENGBERG I. and LUNDBERG A. (1969). An electromyographic
    analysis of muscular activity in the hindlimb of the
    cat during unrestrained locomotion. Acta physiol.
    scand., 75: 614-630.
FELDMAN J.L. (1972). Neural population and motoneurone
    pools. In Abstr. IV Intern.Biophys.Congr. Moscow 1972,
    vol.3, 293-294.
GAMBARJAN P.P., ORLOVSKY G.N., PROTOPOPOVA T.J., SEVE-
    RIN F.V. and SHIK M.L. (1971). The activity of muscles
    during different gaits and adaptive changes of moving
    organs in family Felidae. Morphology and Ecology of
    Vertebrates. Proc.Inst.Zool.Acad.Sci.USSR, 48: 220-
    239 (in Russian)
GANTCHEV G.N., DRAGANOVA N. and DUNEV S. (1972). The
    role of visual information and ocular movements for
    the maintenance of body equilibrium. Agressologie,
    13, B: 55-61.
GRAY J. (1950). The role of peripheral sense organs
    during locomotion in vertebrates. In Physiological
    Mechanisms in Animal Behaviour. Symp.Soc.Exp.Biol.,
    No. 4, 112-126. Cambridge: Univ.Press.
GRILLNER S. (1969). Supraspinal and segmental control
    of static and dynamic gamma-motoneurones in the cat.
    Acta physiol.scand. Suppl. 327: 1-34.
GRILLNER S. and SHIK M.L.(1972). On the deoheading con-
    trol of the lumbosacral spinal cord from the "mesence-
    phalic locomotor region". Acta physiol.scand.(in press).

GROSSMAN R.G.(1958). Effects of stimulation of non-specific thalamic system on locomotor movements in cat. J.
Neurophysiol., 21: 85-93.
GURFINKEL V.S. and ELNER A.M.(1971). Visual control in
equilibrium regulation. In "Visual information processing and Control of Motor Activity". Intern.symp. Sofia.
1969, pp.331-336. Sofia: Publish.Bulg.Acad.Sc.
GURFINKEL V.S., KOTS Y.M., PALTSEV E.I. and FELDMAN A.G.
(1971). The compensation of respiratory disturbances
of the erect posture of man as an example of the organization of interarticular interaction. In Models of
the structural-functional organization of certain biological systems, pp.382-395. Cambridge,Mass.MIT Press.
GURFINKEL V.S., KOTS Y.M. and SHIK M.L.(1965). The regulation of human posture. Moscow, Nauka (in Russian).
HILL D.K.(1968). Tension due to interaction between the
sliding filaments in resting striated muscle.The effect
of stimulation. J.Physiol.(Lond.) 199: 637-684.
HINSEY J.C., RANSON S.W. and McNATTIN R.F.(1930). The
role of the hypothalamus and mesencephalon in locomotion. Arch.Neurol.Psychiat.(Chicago). 23: 1-43.
HONGO Z., JANKOWSKA E. and LUNDBERG A.(1969). The rubro-
spinal tract. Brain Res., 7, 344-364; 365-391.
JANKOWSKA E., JUKES M.G.M., LUND S. and LUNDBERG A.(1967).
The effect of DOPA on the spinal cord. 5. Reciprocal
organization of pathways transmitting excitatory action to alpha motoneurones of flexors and extensors.
Acta physiol.scand., 70: 369-388.
JANKOWSKA E., JUKES M.G.M., LUND S. and LUNDBERG A.(1967).
The effect of DOPA on the spinal cord. 6. Half-center
organization of interneurones transmitting effects
from the flexor reflex afferents. Acta physiol.scand.
70: 389-402.
JANKOWSKA E. and ROBERTS W.J.(1972). An electrophysio-
logical demonstration of the axonal projections of
single spinal interneurones in the cat. J.Physiol.
(Lond.), 222: 597-622.
KULAGIN A.S. and SHIK M.L.(1970). Interaction of sym-
metric extremities during controlled locomotion.
Biofizika, 15: 164-170. (In Russian).
LIPPOLD O.C.I.(1970). Oscillation in the stretch reflex
arc and the origin of the rhithmical,8-12 c/s component
of physiological tremor. J.Physiol.(Lond.),206: 359-392.
LUNDBERG A.(1969). Reflex control of stepping. In The
Nansen Memorial Lecture V.Oslo,Universitetsforlaget.
MAMASAKHLISOV G.V., ELNER A.M. and GURFINKEL V.S.(1972).
Participation of different modality afferentation in
regulation of vertical posture of man. In Abstr.Sec.
Intern.Symp.Motor Control. Varna,1972, p.35 (In Rus-
sian).

MARSHALL J. and WALSH E.G. (1956). Physiological Tremor.
    J.Neurol.Neurosurg.Psychiat., 19: 260-267.
MATTHEWS P.B.C. (1969). Evidence that the secondary as
    well as the primary endings of the muscle spindles
    may be responsible for the tonik stretch reflex of
    the decerebrate cat. J.Physiol.(Lond.), 204: 365-393.
MERTON P.A. (1953). Speculations on the servocontrol of
    movement. In The spinal cord. Ciba Symposium, p.247-
    260, London: Churchill.
MILLER S. (1970). Excitatory and inhibitory proprio-
    spinal pathways from lumbo-sacral to servical seg-
    ments in the cat. Acta physiol.scand., 80: 25A-26A.
NASHNER L.M. (1970). Sensory feed-back in human posture
    control. Thesis. MIT.
NIEUWENHUYS R. (1964). Comparative anatomy of the spin-
    al cord. In Organization of the spinal cord, Progress
    in Brain Res., ed. J.C.Ecceles and J.R.Schadé, vol.11,
    1-57. Amsterdam: Elsevier.
NJIOKIKTJEN Ch. (1972). The influence of vision on the
    vestibulospinal reflex. Agressologie, 13, C, 91-94.
ORLOVSKY G.N. (1970). The activity of reticulospinal
    neurones during locomotion. Biofizika, 15, 728-737.
    (in Russian).
ORLOVSKY G.N. and PAVLOVA G.A. (1972). Vestibular res-
    ponses in neurones of descending pathways during
    locomotion. Neuro-physiologia (Kiev), 4: 311-316. (In
    Russian)
ORLOVSKY G.N., SEVERIN F.V. and SHIK M.L. (1966). The
    influence of speed and load on the coordination of
    movements during the running of the dog. Biofizika,
    11: 364-366. (in Russian)
PHILIPSON M. (1905). L'autonomie et la centralization
    dans le système nerveux des animaux. Travaux du Labor.
    de Physiol.,Inst.Solvay, Bruxelles, 7: 1-208.
ROAF H.E. and SHERRINGTON C.S. (1910). Further remarks
    on the spinal mammalian preparation. Quart. J.Physiol.,
    3: 209-211.
SCHEIBEL M.E. and SCHEIBEL A.B. (1966). Spinal moto-
    neurones, interneurones and Renshaw cells. A Golgi
    study. Archs. ital. Biol., 104: 328-353.
SHAMBES G.M. (1969). Influence of the fusimotor system
    on stance and volitional movement in normal man.
    Am. J. Phys. Med., 48: 225-236.
SHERRINGTON C.S. (1910). Flexion-reflex of the limb,
    crossed extension-reflex and reflex stepping and
    standing. J.Physiol.(Lond.), 40: 28-121.
SHIK M.L. (1971). The controlled locomotion of the
    mesencephalic cat. In Abstr. XXV Intern.Congr.Physiol.
    Sci.,München, vol.8, p.104-105.

SHIK M.L. and ORLOVSKY G.N. (1965). Interlimb coordination during the running of the dog. _Biofizika_, 10:
   1037-1047. (in Russian).
SHIK M.L., ORLOVSKY G,N. and SEVERIN F.V. (1966). The
   organization of locomotor synergy. _Biofizika_, 11:
   879-886. (in Russian).
SHIK M.L., ORLOVSKY G.N. and SEVERIN F.V. (1968). The
   locomotion of a mesencephalic cat elicited by pyramidal stimulation. _Biofizika_, 13: 127-135. (in Russian).
SHIK M.L., SEVERIN F.V. and ORLOVSKY G.N. (1966). The
   control of walking and running by the electrical
   stimulation of the midbrain. _Biofizika_, 11: 659-666.
   (in Russian).
SHIMAMURA M. and LIVINGSTON R.B. (1963). Longitudinal
   conduction systems serving spinal and brain-stem
   coordination. _J.Neurophysiol._, 26: 258-272.
SIROTA M.G. and SHIK M.L. (1972). Cat locomotion induced by stimulation through the elec-rode implanted in
   the midbrain. In _Abstr. IV.Intern.Biophys.Congr._,
   Moscow,1972, vol.4, p.139.
STERLING P. and KNYPERS H.G.J.M. (1968). Anatomical
   organization of the brachial spinal cord of the cat.
   III. The propriospinal connections. _Brain Res._, 7:
   419-443.
SZEKELY G. and CZEH G. (1971). Muscle activities of
   partially innervated limbs during locomotion in
   Ambystoma. _Acta physiol.Acad.Sci.Hung._, 40: 269-286.
TAUB E. and BERMAN A.J. (1968). Movement and learning
   in the absence of sensory feedback. In _The Neuro-_
   psychology of Spatially Oriented Behaviour, ed. S.J.
   Freedmann, p.173-192. Homewood, Ill. Dorsey Press.
TOWER S.S. (1936). Extrapyramidal action from the cat's
   cerebral cortex: motor and inhibitory. _Brain_, 59:
   408-444.
VIALA D. and BUSER P. (1971). Modalités d'obtention
   de rhythmes locomoteurs chez le lapin spinal par
   traitements pharmacologiques. (DOPA, 5-HTP, d-amph-
   étamine). _Brain Res._, 35: 151-165.
WALLER W.H. (1940). Progression movements elicited by
   subthalamic stimulation. _J.Neurophysiol._, 3: 300-307.
WESTMAN J. and BOWSHER D. (1971). The fine structure
   of "non-specific" grey matter (laminae V and VII) in
   the cat spinal cord. _Exp.Brain Res._, 12: 379-388.
WOODS J.W. (1964). Behaviour of chronic decerebrate
   rats. _J.Neurophysiol._, 27: 635-644.

ON THE DYNAMIC EQUILIBRIUM OF THE PEDATAR[x] SYSTEMS

S. V. Fomin and T.I.Stillkind

From the Institute of the Problems of Information Transmission, Acad.Sci.USSR and the
Moscow Physico-Technical Institute

Moscow, USSR

There are certain types of human or animal activities, which, in one way or another, are essentially
connected with use of legs. Besides such kinds of locomotion as walking, jumping and running, they also include non-locomotive movements (standing, marking time,
etc.). Locomotion, on the other hand, includes swimming,
crawling and other types of mechanical displacement in
which the role of legs is not so significant. So considering the types of movement which are impossible without legs, it is convenient to single out as a separate
class all the systems which use legs for their operation.

More rigorously, let us call any system having legs
a pedatar system (PS), if its intrinsic mechanical interaction with the environment, naturally except the gravi-
tavional one, is that occurring through the soles of its
feet, if at all. Arbitrary movements of a PS form a
certain set of pedatar movements.

Two points of this definition should be emphasized.
1°. Besides the "intrinsic mechanical interaction"
there exist other types of interaction, such as resistance of air, random jolts, gusts of wind, etc. However,
this sort of interference is not specifically connected
with pedatar movements and therefore it is not discussed
here.

---

[x] From the Latin pedatus - having legs

2°. Though the physical sense of the situation implies
that contact between the legs and the support is necessary, finite time intervals may exist during which some
of the legs or even all of them are off the support.
The words "if at all" in the definition correspond exactly to such situations.

One of the most important features of the PS is that
the problem of equilibrium is of special significance
for any such system. All types of pedatar movements can
be effected only if equilibrium is preserved in the
process. It should also be noted that the problem of
maintaining equilibrium of a PS is by no means trivial,
since most natural PS are rather unstable statically,
and to keep stable a PS must possess a sophisticated
control system.

It is to be noted besides, that the requirements of
static stability of a system and its mobility might be
called contradictory.

If for fast movement the legs should be light, have
considerable length, with small momenta of inertia,
statically it is more advantageous for a PS to have
short, solid legs, thus bringing the center of gravity
closer to the ground. Nature seems to solve its problems
having found a compromise in such a way that stable
equilibrium of a PS is possible only because of the
existence of a rather subtle control system.

The functional features are in many respects responsible for the structure and properties of the PS.
Thus, any PS must contain a structure which handles the
selection of the movement task; a structure which controls the motion while the system is solving this task;
and, of course, the mechanical structure 'per se'. It
goes without saying that both the formulation of the
movement task and its realisation are secured by control
but analysing the solution of the given movement task we
see that the control functions are performed by a second
structure, which we shall call for brevity a control
structure.

It is evident that in studying the control patterns
of a PS a deeper insight into the mechanical structure
of a PS is necessary as it affects profoundly the
organization and functioning of the control system as a
whole. In fact, any movement task can be reduced to a
change or stabilization of a state of the mechanical
structure, and this is what control is responsible for.

At the same time the control system in any pedatar movement should also maintain the equilibrium of the PS; The
system can not be defined as pedatar if its equilibrium
is lost.

Before proceeding, the concept of equilibrium should
be defined. Note that in this case the definition cannot be based on the classical theory of the stability,
which insists heavily on the behaviour of a system at
$t \rightarrow \infty$. The matter is that the control structure of a PS
has considerable freedom in selecting a control mode,
which results in the fact that no state of the system at
$t = t_o$ can guarantee its equilibrium at $t \rightarrow \infty$. Therefore, in principle, a PS can be thought of as being in
equilibrium at t_o if a possibility exists that it will
not fall at $t > t_o$. Now let us introduce some basic
definitions.

The mechanical state of a PS or, briefly, a state,
is by definition, any set of independent kinematic
variables, which completely determine the position and
velocities of the PS in a fixed coordinate system. The
values of the variables selected are the components of
a vector X in the phase space X of the PS.

The driving efforts that are physiologically possible
for the organism involved define a region V which is
bounded in the space W of all control modes. In order
for a system to be pedatar a certain specific sub-region
$U \subset V$ is required which will be called the region of
pedatar control modes. In other words, the region of
pedatar control modes is precisely the region of control
modes that are allowed for the PS.

Any trajectory $\Gamma \subset W$ is called a control mode,
which in the process of motion is described by the
control vector $u(t)$. Then the control mode Γ is pedatar
if $\Gamma \subset U$.

Let X be the phase space of an arbitrary PS. We
shall say that the point $x_1 \in X$ is accessible from the
point $x_o \in X$ if there exists a pedatar control mode,
which transfers the PS from x_o to x_1 i.e. if for any t_o
there exist $t_1 > t_o$ and $\Gamma \subset U$ such that $x(t_o) = x_o$ and
$x(t_1) = x_1$. The largest region $M \subset X$ which has the property
that any two of its points are mutually accessible,will
be called the region of reversibility of the PS.

Then, by definition, the PS is in equilibrium at

$t=t_o$ if its state is in the region of reversibility at
$t=t_o$ i.e. if $x(t_o) \in M$. In this case there exists at
least one pedatar control mode that will prevent the
system from falling.

Two points here deserve special discussion.
1. There can be several reversibility regions for a
PS, their total number being determined by the mechanical structure of the PS and its region of pedatar control
modes. It should be pointed out, however, that in all
cases of practical interest the reversibility region is
either unique, or a certain region can naturally be
singled out among the available ones, with the task of
equilibrium to be solved for the region thus selected.

2. The above definition holds for a PS of arbitrary
mechanical structure; in particular, it is valid for a
PS having any number of legs. No doubt, the fewer legs
a PS has, the more vital for it is the problem of maintaining equilibrium.

Let us now consider the reversibility region in connection with the motion control organization. The PS
control system should obviously keep all phase trajectories within the reversibility region, since crossing its
boundary will inevitably result in falling. The requirement of equilibrium is thus a constraint on the phase
trajectories of the system.

As a rule, there is no need to deal with the whole
of the reversibility region in solving the movement task.
Moreover, it might be unreasonable. This is substantiat-
ed by the fact that keeping the state of a PS close to
the boundary of the reversibility region usually requires
a considerable control drive, which may turn costly in
terms even of energy spent.

Besides, there is a variety of usually unpredictable
disturbances acting on a PS under natural conditions. If
the disturbance is strong enough the state vector may
cross the boundary of the reversibility region. Friction
uncertainly may also result in a fall of a PS if the
exact value of the friction coefficient at the point of
contact is not known in advance.

However, due to the importance of the problem of
equilibrium, its solution should be rather reliable. This
is why the phase trajectories of a system must not pass
too close to the boundary of the reversibility region,
so that the control structure should have both time and

driving power, if necessary, to keep the system in equilibrium. Here the distance, properly defined, between
the state of a PS and the boundary of its reversibility
region can serve as an estimate of the stability margin
of the PS.

Each movement task, as a rule, brings into play additional constraints either on the region of pedatar
control modes or on the system's trajectories. If the
movement task does not prevent the PS from maintaining
the equilibrium, the constraints bring about shrinking
of the original reversibility region to a sub-region,
containing all phase trajectories which correspond to
solutions of a given movement task. The fact that the
state vector of a PS may leave this sub-region means
a failure of the system to accomplish the task but does
not lead to a fall if the state is still inside the
reversibility region.

In a typical movement the state of a system is kept
in the reversibility region not too close to its boundary. The trajectories in such cases can be chosen from
a wide variety, for the particular reasons of selecting
specific trajectories may vary. There is no exception
to this: if there is a risk that the system may fall,
i.e. the state of the PS passes close to the boundary of
the reversibility region, the maintenance of equilibrium
acquires top priority and the control structure tries
to reverse the state from the dangerous zone, even if
this contradicts the movement task.

Mathematical description of real pedatar systems
(man, animal, robot) is a rather complicated job. As an
illustration of the concepts given above we shall now
consider the simple two-link model of the vertical
posture of man. This model is shown in Fig. 1.

It consists of two rigid links, which simulate the
feet and trunk of a man. The links are joined to each
other by an ideal hinge, with the axis perpendicular to
the plane of the figure.

The momentum u of internal forces which act in the
hinge is the control of the system. The control u is
selected by the system arbitrarily, provided the natural
constraint $(u) \leqslant \tilde{u}$ is satisfied, where $\tilde{u} > 0$ is some constant.

The foot is at rest on an ideal support and there
is no slipping.

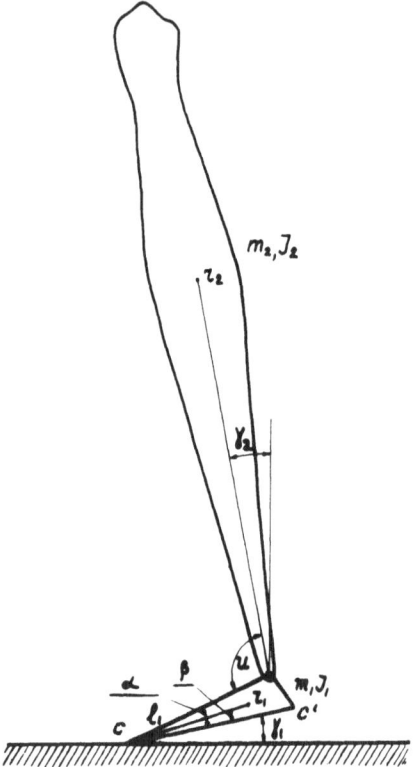

<u>Fig. 1</u>   Simple two-link model of the vertical posture of
        man.

     We consider only such situations when the support
comes into contact with point c , point c′ or both, and
in these cases the system will be said to stand on its
toe, heel and foot respectively. The equations of motion of the model for each of these situations are,
generally speaking, different, but can easily be derived one from another. Assume, for example, that the
system stands on its toe. We have the following two
equations of motion:

$$(y_1 + m_2 l_1^2)\ddot{\gamma}_1 - m_2 l_1 r_2 \left[\ddot{\gamma}_2 \sin(\gamma_1 + \gamma_2 + \alpha) + \dot{\gamma}_2^2 \cos(\gamma_1 + \gamma_2 + \alpha)\right] +$$

$$+ m_1 g r_1 \cos(\gamma_1 + \beta) + m_2 g l_1 \cos(\gamma_1 + \alpha) = u \qquad (1)$$

$$y_2 \ddot{\gamma}_2 - m_2 l_1 r_2 \left[\ddot{\gamma}_1 \sin(\gamma_1 + \gamma_2 + \alpha) + \dot{\gamma}_1^2 \cos(\gamma_1 + \gamma_2 + \alpha)\right] -$$

$$- m_2 g r_2 \sin\gamma_2 = u \qquad (2)$$

For the system standing on the heel the equations of motion are obtained from Eqs.(1)-(2) by the substitutions $\gamma_1 \to \pi - \gamma_1$, $\gamma_2 \to -\gamma_2$ and, of course,

$$y_1 \to y_1'; \quad r_1 \to r_1'; \quad l_1 \to l_1'; \quad \alpha \to \alpha'; \quad \beta \to \beta';$$

Let us look more closely into the third of the cases mentioned above, namely, when the whole foot is in contact with the support. It is to this particular case that the following discussion is devoted.

The equations of motion of the system are then given by Eqs. (1)-(2) with $\gamma_1(t) \equiv 0$. The following form of the equation of motion is obtained from Eq. (2).

$$y_2 \ddot{\gamma}_2 - m_2 g r_2 \sin \gamma_2 = u \qquad (2')$$

while Eq. (1) gives

$$-m_2 l_1 r_2 \left[\ddot{\gamma}_2 \sin(\gamma_2 + \alpha) + \dot{\gamma}_2^2 \cos(\gamma_2 + \alpha) \right] - m_1 g r_1 \cos \beta + \qquad (1')$$
$$+ m_2 g l_1 \cos \alpha = u$$

The angle γ_1 cannot become negative due to the resulting support's reaction momentum. There is no need to introduce this angle explicitly in the equations; its contribution is obtained by letting Eq.(1') become an inequality, with u being less or equal to the left-hand term. Substitution into Eq. (1') of the expression for $\ddot{\gamma}_2$ obtained from Eq. (2') yields:

$$u \left[1 - \frac{m_2 l_1 r_2}{y_2} \sin(\gamma_2 + \alpha) \right] \leq m_1 g r_1 \cos\beta + m_2 g l_1 \cos \alpha - \qquad (3)$$
$$- \frac{(m_2 r_2)^2}{y_2} g l_1 \sin(\gamma_2 + \alpha) - m_2 l_1 r_2 \dot{\gamma}_2^2 \cos(\gamma_2 + \alpha);$$

Since $l_1 < r_2$ the expression $1 + \dfrac{m_2 l_1 r_2}{y_2} \cdot \sin(\gamma_2 + \alpha)$ is easily seen to be positive for all values of γ_2. After some elementary transformations we obtain

$$u \leq \frac{b \cos(2\gamma_2 + \alpha) - c \dot{\gamma}_2^2 \cos(\gamma_2 + \alpha) + d}{1 + a \sin(\gamma_2 + \alpha)} \overset{\Delta}{=} Q_+ (\gamma_2, \dot{\gamma}_2) \qquad (3')$$

where the following notations are introduced:

$$c \overset{\Delta}{=} m_2 l_1 r_2 ; \qquad a \overset{\Delta}{=} \frac{c}{y_2} ; \qquad b \overset{\Delta}{=} \frac{1}{2} a m_2 g r_2 ;$$

$$d \overset{\Delta}{=} m_1 g r_1 \cos\beta + m_2 g l_1 \cos\alpha \left(1 - \frac{m_2 r_2^2}{2 y_2}\right) ;$$

Thus the original equations are reduced to just one equation of motion (2') with the control restriction given by Eq. (3'). The physical sense of this restriction is that at $\gamma_1(0) = \dot{\gamma}_1(0) = 0$ the heel is unable to break away from the support , which is exactly the condition for the existence of solutions of Eqs. (1)-(2) with $\gamma_1(t) \equiv 0$.

However, a similar condition holds for the toe if the system is to stand on the whole foot

$$u \geqslant -\frac{b'\cos(2\gamma_2 - \alpha') - c'\dot{\gamma}_2^2 \cos(\gamma_2 - \alpha') + d'}{1 - a'\sin(\gamma_2 - \alpha')} \overset{\Delta}{=} Q\,(\gamma_2, \dot{\gamma}_2) \qquad (3'')$$

(the notations here are obvious).

Thus for the model to be able to stand, the whole foot being in contact with the support, the following double inequality is to hold:

$$Q_-(\gamma_2, \dot{\gamma}_2) \leqslant u \leqslant Q_+(\gamma_2, \dot{\gamma}_2) ; \qquad (4)$$

The condition given by this equation becomes sufficient if the initial conditions $\gamma_1(0) = \dot{\gamma}_1(0) = 0$ are taken into account.

Naturally it is necessary that $Q_-(\gamma_2, \dot{\gamma}_2) \leqslant Q_+(\gamma_2, \dot{\gamma}_2)$

This condition is non-trivial in the general case, e.g. it is easily seen to be violated at large $\dot{\gamma}_2$. It holds, however, for those ranges of angles and velocities, containing the point (0,0), in which we are interested.

Inequality (4) turns out to be more restrictive than $|u| \leqslant \tilde{u}$ if the mechanical parameters of the model are approaching those of man. This, though not rigorously, follows from the fact that man can easily lift a heel or a toe from the floor while the position of his body is practically unchanged,

Eq. (2') and inequality (4) actually simplify, to some extent, the original model. The simplified model will briefly be referred to as the F-model.

Now, for the F-model, let us consider a problem of constructing its reversibility region M, which is the largest region of the phase space $X = \{\gamma_2, \dot{\gamma}_2\}$ in which the phase point of the F-model can stay infinitely long.

Let us first find the region S of static stability of our model. This region obviously is a segment of the straight line $\dot{\gamma}_2 = 0$:

$$S = \left\{ \gamma_2, \dot{\gamma}_2 : {}^*\gamma < \gamma_2 < \gamma^*, \ \dot{\gamma}_2 = 0 \right\}$$

The boundary values ${}^*\gamma$ and γ^* can be determined from the following conditions

$$Q_+({}^*\gamma, 0) = -m_2 gr_2 \sin {}^*\gamma \tag{5}$$

$$Q_-(\gamma^*, 0) = -m_2 gr_2 \sin \gamma^* \tag{5'}$$

Actually. Eqs. (5) and (5') guarantee that the system's center of gravity stays within the limits of the support contour.

It is quite obvious, however, that if $\dot{\gamma}_2$ is different from zero, the condition ${}^*\gamma \leq \gamma_2 \leq \gamma^*$ is by no means sufficient for the equilibrium of the F-model. Even more, it is not sufficient at $\dot{\gamma}_2 = 0$ either, because in this case the system has complete freedom of selecting a control mode. Let us recall that we are looking for a region for which at least one allowed control mode exists making the phase point stay in it at all moments of time.

Two boundaries of the reversibility region are easily seen to be given by the solutions of the equation of motion of the F-model determined by the conditions:

$$\begin{cases} u = Q_-(\gamma_2, \dot{\gamma}) \\ \gamma_2(0) = \gamma^* - 0 \quad (\tilde{m}_1) \\ \dot{\gamma}_2(0) = 0 \end{cases} \quad \text{and} \quad \begin{cases} u = Q_+(\gamma_2, \dot{\gamma}_2) \\ \gamma_2(0) = {}^*\gamma + 0 \quad (\tilde{m}_2) \\ \dot{\gamma}_2(0) = 0 \end{cases}$$

Numerical integration on a digital computer has been carried out to find these solutions, which is apparently the simplest way of obtaining them.

The other two boundary lines are given by the solutions of Eq.(2') determined by the conditions

$$\begin{cases} u = Q_-(\gamma_2, \dot{\gamma}_2) \\ \gamma_2(T) = \gamma^*{-}0 \quad (m_1) \\ \dot{\gamma}_2(T) = 0 \end{cases} \quad \text{and} \quad \begin{cases} u = Q_+(\gamma_2, \dot{\gamma}_2) \\ \gamma_2(T) = {}^*\gamma + 0 \quad (m_2) \\ \dot{\gamma}_2(T) = 0 \end{cases}$$

where $T > 0$ is a certain time moment, which is not known in advance.

Since equations of mechanics are invariant under the time reversal transformation, it is clear that the last two curves can be obtained from $\tilde{m}_1$ and $\tilde{m}_2$ by substituting $\dot{\gamma}_2 \rightarrow -\dot{\gamma}_2$ so that only $\tilde{m}_1$ and $\tilde{m}_2$ have to be computed.

The reversibility region for the F-model having thus been constructed, a particular way of stabilizing (an algorithm of control) the model can be selected (Fig.2).

In general, there is a variety of algorithms which may be used for keeping equilibrium. Their only common feature is that control modes $u = Q_-(\gamma_2, \dot{\gamma}_2)$ and $u = Q_+(\gamma_2, \dot{\gamma}_2)$ should be activated whenever the phase point of the system comes into contact with the boundaries m_1 and m_2 respectively.

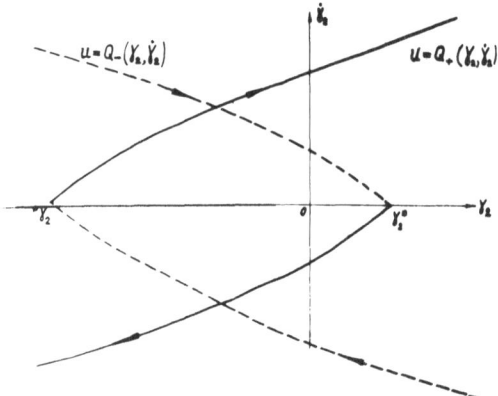

Fig. 2. A possible algorithm of control for the F-model.

This is the necessary condition of stability: equilibrium is lost as soon as the system crosses m_1 or m_2 .
The role of the m_1 and m_2 trajectories themselves is
to switch the control modes. As for selecting the control
mode $u(\gamma_2, \dot{\gamma}_2)$ in the reversibility region proper, it
should not contradict the condition given by Eq. (4).

So far we have assumed that there is no external
perturbation. Suppose now that some noise μ interferes
with the F-model. Let the perturbation have the dimen-
sion of the momentum of forces and be represented in
the equations by the terms additive with u . The disturbance can result therefore both from environmental
action and from control failures. There can, of course,
be no equilibrium if the value of μ is too large. It is
therefore reasonable to assume that μ is bounded:

$$|\mu| \leqslant \delta$$

where the constant $\delta > 0$ is not too large.

Let us consider the case of the greatest hazard for
the system, when only the estimate of disturbance is
known, the noise being unpredictable and its level not
being registered by the system accurately (i.e. only
the value of δ and information on the phase coordinates
of the system are used for control). We shall demonstrate
that it is possible to keep the equilibrium of the F-
model under such conditions.

Thus we have $|\mu| \leqslant \delta$. Inequality (4) in this case
takes the form

$$Q_- + \delta \leqslant u \leqslant Q_+ - \delta \qquad\qquad (6)$$

(The control constraints have thus become more stringent.
In fact, if for example $u(t) = u^*$ and $Q_- + \delta \leqslant u^* \leqslant Q_+$
then a disturbance of the level $\mu = +\delta$ leads to instant
breaking of contact between the foot and the support,
i.e. to a loss of equilibrium of the F-model.)

It will be noted that the concept of static stability itself loses much of its sense in the presence of
noise. Maintenance of equilibrium becomes fundamentally
a dynamic problem. On a purely formal basis, however,
one could define the region: $S_{2\delta} \subset S$

$$S_{2\delta} = \left\{ \gamma_2, \dot{\gamma}_2 : \,^*\gamma_{2\delta} \leqslant \gamma_2 \leqslant \gamma_{2\delta}{}^*, \dot{\gamma}_2 = 0 \right\}$$

Here $^*\gamma_{2\delta}$ and $\gamma_{2\delta}{}^*$ are determined by the following two relations:

$$Q_+(\,^*\gamma_{2\delta},0) - 2\delta = -m_2 g r_2 \sin \,^*\gamma_{2\delta}$$

$$Q_-(\gamma_{2\delta}{}^*,0) + 2\delta = -m_2 g r_2 \sin \gamma_{2\delta}{}^*$$

The necessary condition $^*\gamma_{2\delta} < \gamma_{2\delta}{}^*$ is sure to be satisfied if

$$\delta < \frac{1}{4} \min \left\{ Q_+(\gamma,\dot{\gamma}) - Q_-(\gamma,\dot{\gamma}) \right\}$$

$$\{\gamma, \dot{\gamma}\} \in M$$

Consider two more control switch lines, which are mirror images with respect to $\dot{\gamma}_2 = 0$ axis of the solution of Eq. (2') defined by the conditions

$$\begin{cases} u = Q_- + 2\delta \\ \gamma_2(0) = \gamma_{2\delta}{}^* - 0 \quad (m_{1\delta}) \\ \dot{\gamma}_2(0) = 0 \end{cases} \quad \text{and} \quad \begin{cases} u = Q_+ - 2\delta \\ \gamma_2(0) = \,^*\gamma_{2\delta} + 0 \quad (m_{2\delta}) \\ \dot{\gamma}_2(0) = 0 \end{cases}$$

Here only two conditions affect the choice of the control algorithm:

a) control modes $u = Q_- + \delta$ and $u = Q_+ - \delta$ are activated on the control switch lines $m_{1\delta}$ and $m_{2\delta}$ respectively;

b) control should satisfy inequality (6) in the area external to $m_{1\delta}$ and $m_{2\delta}$. The F-model is stable if we have $\{\gamma_2(0), \dot{\gamma}_2(0)\} \in S_{2\delta}$ as well.

The conditions a) and b), to be sure, allow for specific improvements of the control algorithm. which can be realized in many ways; however, their character of necessity should be emphasized: if any of these conditions is violated, a disturbance can be found which makes the phase point leave the reversibility region.

Below two examples of effective algorithms are given. The following algorithm is perhaps the simplest one. Assume that $\{\gamma_2(0), \dot{\gamma}_2(0)\} \in S_{2\delta}$. Under the control

$u = Q_+ - \delta$ the system is moving until it crosses the control switch line $m_{1\delta}$. Then the control $u = Q_- + \delta$ is activated, and the system is moving until it meets the line $m_{2\delta}$. The control $u = Q_+ - \delta$ takes over at that stage, etc.

It can easily be verified that a controlled model of this sort is stable even though it is known about the possible perturbations only that they are within certain limits, with the absolute value smaller than or equal to δ . Of course, this situation diminishes the region of the system's motion in the absence of per- turbations (when disturbances may or may not occur). But this is the price to be paid for stability.

Let us now describe the second control algorithm. Take the point $\{\tilde{\gamma}, 0\}$ which is, in a certain sense, the "central" point of the reversibility region. Here $\tilde{\gamma}$ may be taken equal, say to $\frac{1}{2}({}^*\gamma_{2\delta} + \gamma_{2\delta}{}^*)$. Take then a time- independent control mode $u^\circ = -m_2 g r_2 \sin \tilde{\gamma}$, the point $\tilde{\gamma}$ thus becoming a position of the unstable equilibrium of the F-model at $u = u^\circ$. Now let us introduce two more control switch lines: these lines will be the solutions of Eq.(2') defined by the conditions:

$$\begin{cases} u = u^\circ \\ \gamma_2(0) = \tilde{\gamma} - 0 \quad (m_{10}) \\ \dot{\gamma}_2(0) = 0 \end{cases} \quad \text{and} \quad \begin{cases} u = u^\circ \\ \gamma_2(0) = \tilde{\gamma} + 0 \quad (m_{20}) \\ \dot{\gamma}_2(0) = 0 \end{cases}$$

and subsequently reflected with respect to the $\dot{\gamma}_2 = 0$ axis (Fig.3).

Assume that ${}^*\gamma_{2\delta} < \gamma_2(0) < \gamma_{2\delta}{}^*$. The system starts mov- ing under the control $u = Q_+ - \delta$. When the control switch line m_{10} is crossed, the control mode $u = u^\circ$ is activated, making the phase point approach the point $\{\tilde{\gamma}, 0\}$. However, since this position or equilibrium is instable, the system sooner or later will reach $m_{1\delta}$ or $m_{2\delta}$ with im- mediate activation of the control mode $u = Q_- + \delta$ (on $m_{1\delta}$) or $u = Q_+ - \delta$ (on $m_{2\delta}$). The proper control mode operated until the next crossing of the m_{10} or m_{20} trajectories, where once again the control mode $u = u^\circ$ is activated.

This scheme of control seems to be more reasonable. In fact, sizable control effort is necessary only when the system comes close to the boundary of the reversibil- ity region, i.e. when the risk of falling is great; at all other times control effort is close to being

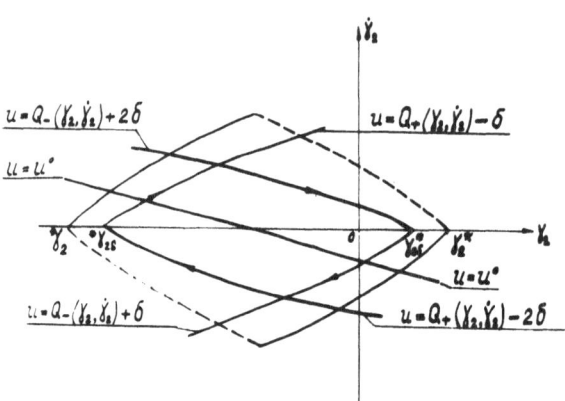

Fig. 3.

negligible. But the latter algorithm is somewhat more
complicated than the former. One could of course suggest
more advanced control schemes by making them more sophisticated. However, the possibility of solving the
equilibrium problem by using simple technique seems to
be attractive.

Of special interest is the behaviour of a model with
delays in its feedback control loop.

To start with, we shall consider the problem of un-
perturbed motion assuming that control effort at time t
is determined by the state of the system at time $t-\tau$,
i.e. by $\gamma_2(t-\tau)$ and $\dot{\gamma}_2(t-\tau)$. The equation of motion
of the F-model now takes the form:

$$y_2\ddot{\gamma}_2(t) - m_2 g r_2 \sin \gamma_2(t) = u\left[\gamma_2(t-\tau), \dot{\gamma}_2(t-\tau)\right] \qquad (2'')$$

Eq. (2'') is a delay differential equation. As is
known a solution of an equation of this type does exist
and is unique if the function $\gamma_2(t)$ and its derivative
$\dot{\gamma}_2(t)$ are known at all points of a certain initial segment of the length τ e.g. of the segment $[-\tau, 0]$.

On the basis of the idea of control switch lines it
is not difficult to develop an algorithm, which stabil-
izes the F-model, provided, of course, that the value
of τ is sufficiently small compared with the time of
control-free motion of the system from the center of
the reversibility region to its boundary. It is clear

that in this case, as before, the following inequality
should be satisfied for each phase trajectory of the
system:

$$Q_-[\gamma_2(t), \dot{\gamma}_2(t)] \leq u(t) \leq Q_+[\gamma_2(t), \dot{\gamma}_2(t)] \qquad (4')$$

Some differences may arise now in ensuring the fulfilment of condition (4'), since we assume that only
information about the state of the system at time $t - \tau$
is available at time t. In the absence of random disturbances information on the state of the system before
time $t - \tau$ makes it possible to determine the system's
state at time t (e.g. by solving Eq.(2") . On the other
hand, if random disturbances are bounded, with the constant δ as their upper bound, the construction of stabil-
ity-oriented control algorithms can be reduced to eval-
uating the least favourable situations, switching control modes on such phase trajectories which pass far
enough from the boundary of the reversibility region to
ensure that in all cases the system does not leave it.

Control algorithms, which are basically similar to
algorithms 1) and 2) constructed for delay-free systems,
can be developed in this way.

I N D E X